# CLASSIFICATION OF NEUROSIS

**Peter Tyrer, MD, MRCP, FRCPsych**

Senior Lecturer and Consultant Psychiatrist,
St Charles' Hospital, London

JOHN WILEY & SONS

Chichester · New   York · Brisbane · Toronto · Singapore

Copyright © 1989 by John Wiley & Sons Ltd.
Baffins Lane, Chichester
West Sussex PO19 1UD, England

Distributed in the United States of America,
Canada and Japan by Alan R. Liss, Inc.,
41 East 11th Street, New York,
NY 10003, USA.

*Other Wiley Editorial Offices*

John Wiley & Sons, Inc., 605 Third Avenue,
New York, NY 10158-0012, USA

Jacaranda Wiley Ltd, G.P.O. Box 859, Brisbane,
Queensland 4001, Australia

John Wiley & Sons (Canada) Ltd, 22 Worcester Road,
Rexdale, Ontario M9W 1L1, Canada

John Wiley & Sons (SEA) Pte Ltd, 37 Jalan Pemimpin 05-04,
Block B, Union Industrial Building, Singapore 2057

*Library of Congress Cataloging-in-Publication Data*

Tyrer, Peter J.
    Classification of neurosis / Peter Tyrer.
        p.   cm.
    Bibliography: p.
    Includes index.
    ISBN 0 471 91777 X
    1. Neuroses—Classification.   I. Title.
    [DNLM: 1. Neurotic Disorders—classification.   WM 15 T992c]
RC530.T97   1989
616.85'2'0012—dc20
DNLM/DLC
for Library of Congress                                    89-9200
                                                              CIP

*British Library Cataloguing in Publication Data*

Tyrer, Peter, 1940–
    Classification of neurosis.
    1. Man. Neurosis
    I. Title
    616.85'2

    ISBN 0 471 91777 X

Typeset by Inforum Typesetting, Portsmouth
Printed and bound by Biddles Ltd, Guildford

# CLASSIFICATION
# OF NEUROSIS

*For Jonathan, Clare and Freya*

# Contents

Foreword ........................................................ ix

Preface ......................................................... xi

Prologue ........................................................ xv

Chapter 1 Neurosis and the International
          Classification of Diseases ........................... 1

Chapter 2 Neurosis: The American Perspective .................. 13

Chapter 3 Panic and Generalized Anxiety Disorder ............. 17

Chapter 4 Phobic and Obsessional Disorders ................... 42

Chapter 5 Depressive Disorders ............................... 63

Chapter 6 Somatoform and Dissociative Disorders .............. 87

Chapter 7 Stress and Adjustment Disorders ................... 118

Chapter 8 General Neurotic Syndrome and Mixed
          Anxiety–Depressive Disorders ...................... 132

Bibliography ................................................. 165

Index ....................................................... 186

# Foreword

Books which are primarily concerned with the implications of classifications of psychiatric disorders have always been less common than new classifications themselves. This is unfortunate, because all classifications, including those which aspire to being 'atheoretical', embody many fundamental assumptions about the nature of their subject matter. They also have a major influence on how their users conceptualise the phenomena in question. Indeed, this may well be why new typologies appear so frequently, for those who are persuaded to adopt them will also, wittingly or unwittingly, adopt most of their authors' underlying assumptions. Treatises devoted to the classification of neuroses are particularly uncommon. It is generally assumed that the classification of psychotic disorders or of depressive illnesses is more important, and also that these topics can be more profitably discussed because more relevant empirical evidence is available. This book is therefore as unusual as it is welcome.

Dr Tyrer describes what will be for the next decade or so the two most influential and widely used classifications of neurotic disorders—the forthcoming (10th) revision of the International Classification of Disease (ICD-10) and the American Psychiatric Association's classifications DSM-III and DSM-III-R. He focuses on the differences between them and the novel concepts, like Panic Disorder, which are common to both. He also discusses the implications of these differences and the relevant empirical evidence—the clinical trials, family studies and follow-up studies—that help to

ix

establish or to undermine the validity of the diagnostic concepts concerned. He therefore not only describes the phenomena of neurotic illness and contemporary classifications of these phenomena; he also raises important practical and theoretical questions that might otherwise have remained unasked.

Dr Tyrer writes as a practising clinician, observing as he does so, with only the faintest hint of menace, that as 'the fate of any classification depends on the reaction of its main users it is clinicians who hold the key to success'. This stance is one of this book's greatest strengths, for it is apparent in every chapter that the text has been written by someone who combines a comprehensive knowledge of the literature with extensive personal experience of the symptomatology, treatment and prognosis of neurotic disorders. Dr Tyrer has, of course, prejudices of his own. He remains convinced that 'neurosis' is still a valuable concept, that different clinical presentations are less discrete and stable than the architects of DSM-III have assumed, that new concepts should not be adopted until they have been validated by long-term follow-up studies, and that patients with a fluctuating mélange of depressive, anxious and obsessional symptoms are so common that the term 'general neurotic syndrome' must be retained to describe them. Several experienced psychiatrists already share these views; others will be converted to them by reading this important monograph.

R.E. KENDELL
Department of Psychiatry
Edinburgh University
May, 1989

# Preface

There has been great interest in classifying psychiatric disorders in the past decade. Much of this has been stimulated by the introduction of the third edition of the *Diagnostic and Statistical Manual of Mental Disorders* (more familiarly known as DSM-III) by the American Psychiatric Association in 1980. The *International Classification of Diseases* (ICD) of the World Health Organization has also shown major reforms and stimulated more interest in the diagnostic process. One of the main subjects of reform has been neurosis. Whereas in previous classifications the neuroses have been prominent in the description of all so-called 'minor' psychiatric disorders they have largely been renamed and reformulated in the latest classifications.

This is a major change and one that should not be allowed to pass without comment. Much argument has gone on behind the closed doors of the committees of classification but relatively little has been aired amongst a wider audience. This book attempts to remedy this. My viewpoint is primarily that of a clinician. As ultimately the fate of any classification depends on the reaction of its main users it is clinicians who hold the key to success of the new systems. This is not to decry the great contribution made by research workers in developing and nurturing the sometimes fragile concepts embodied in new developments, and also the advantages of better formulation of diagnostic description in research studies, but a classification that is only useful in research is unlikely to survive.

A format consistent with the clinical approach is used throughout this book. After introductory chapters outlining the concepts behind the DSM and ICD classifications the main conditions formerly subsumed under the neuroses are described. The DSM and ICD descriptions are compared and discussed, and the reasoning behind the reformulation is described. Case histories are given to highlight the use of the classifications in practice and these are followed by a critique of the diagnosis under four headings: its clarity of description, the amount of overlap with other disorders, its stability measured through studies of outcome, and treatment implications. In the final chapter the shortcomings of the classifications are examined and suggestions made as to how they can be overcome.

In the American classification, DSM, individual disorders are described using the upper case. Because they are referred to so frequently in this book and because the same convention does not always apply to the diagnoses in ICD all diagnoses are given in the lower case throughout this book.

Classifications are derived by consensus determined by negotiation. The final result is sometimes lop-sided, best summarised as the saying, 'a camel is a horse designed by a committee'. A single author has no such handicap but is much more affected by personal bias. I should like to delude myself that this has been kept to a minimum in the following pages but know this cannot be true. My belief that the concept of neurosis is a good one for clinical practice, and has more substance than the new classifications imply, will be obvious to anyone reading beyond the first pages. All good words attract meanings they did not originally possess; neurosis may have attracted too many but when stripped of its redundant trimmings still informs and describes better than any of its replacements.

I am particularly grateful to the World Health Organization for permission to quote from the 1988 draft of the tenth revision of Chapter V of the _International Classification of Diseases_, Categories F00-F99, 'Mental, behavioural and developmental disorders: clinical descriptions and diagnostic guidelines', produced by the Division of Mental Health, Geneva. The draft is provisional and is intended to be published in 1990 and released for general use in 1992. The copyright for the trial drafts is held by the World Health Organization and any information from them repeated in this book should not be reproduced without their permission. I am also grateful to the American Psychiatric Association for permission to quote from the third edition and revised third edition of DSM, published in 1980 and 1987 respectively.

Finally I should like to thank all my colleagues who have provided constant stimulation by either arguing against or agreeing with my views on the classification of neurosis, and particularly including Patricia Casey, Allen Frances, Robert Kendell, Alan Kerr, Donald

Klein, Eugene Paykel, Sir Martin Roth and David Sheehan, and to acknowledge my debt to the late William Sargant and Eliot Slater for first showing me that the subject was important in clinical practice. Bonnie Lucas, Margaret O'Mahoney and my wife, Ann, have been invaluable secretarial assistants and Mike Taylor has provided essential library skills. Any errors in the following pages would be multiplied tenfold but for their vigilance.

PETER TYRER
London
November, 1988

# Prologue

Mrs Green was 36 and had just been referred by her general practitioner to a new psychiatrist. She felt ashamed of herself for not being able to 'pull herself together' as her mother had constantly advised her throughout her life. She had never known what it was like to be 'together' and when advised from an early age to 'snap out of it' was far from clear whether 'it' was thought to be something she had made up or allowed to develop through lack of will. Many times she had been told she was 'neurotic' but she was not sure whether this was a statement of fact or a personal criticism. To her the word meant very little but she had learnt that it was never said sympathetically and was normally used when others were irritated or angry with her. It also tended to be used about her when she saw doctors although, for some reason she could not understand, it was never said to her directly. She dreaded seeing new doctors because they made her feel inadequate and vulnerable. They used to spend several minutes going through her file before talking to her about her latest problems and she often heard them sighing while they were reading.

Although she understood the concept of a 'nervous breakdown' she could not really use it to describe herself. To have a breakdown you had to be able to compare it with a time of 'nervous health' and she could not remember such a time in her life since the birth of consciousness. She seemed to be in a state of continuous breakdown; it was as though her nerves had not been made right in the first place rather than going wrong at a later date. It always upset her when doctors asked her when her problem first started because it did not seem to have a start or an end; it was always with her and the doctors' insistence on matching it up with events in her life seemed to be artificial.

When seen in the clinic she gave her usual account of feeling 'a continuous bag of nerves' that had become much worse recently. She realised in giving this account that she was not being entirely truthful as she kept on stressing how much worse she had been recently and how financial and domestic worries had provoked this. She was putting across the idea of nervous breakdown to the doctor because of past experience that it was more likely to be taken seriously and her present feelings considered sympathetically. Because of these recent worries she admitted that she was quite unable to carry out even a simple task at home and that her husband and two children had been forced to take over from her.

The new doctor was also puzzled. Although Mrs Green related her symptoms to stresses it was difficult to decide when these symptoms had started as direct enquiry showed they had been present to some degree since the age of 7. At that time she had become frightened and refused to go to school. Eventually she had been referred to a child guidance clinic when she developed ideas that parts of her body were shrinking and that it was unsafe to sit on a chair in case she was electrocuted. The only time she had shown anything approaching normal mental function was for about two years between the time she left home and when she married at the age of 20. She was aware that her father was a similarly nervous person and had long periods away from work because he could not cope with responsibilities there. From him she developed the idea that some people were born nervous and it was a cross she would have to bear throughout her life.

Her marriage was a strain at first because of all the unsettling changes that followed but her ability to cope suffered most after the birth of their first son. A year later she became anxious, depressed and fearful and was referred to a psychiatrist. He confidently made a diagnosis of depressive illness and treated her with electroconvulsive therapy as an outpatient. She was also treated with antidepressants (amitriptyline) and improved to some extent. Nevertheless, she remained under constant strain and after the birth of an unplanned second child 18 months later she was referred to a different psychiatrist. He noted that she was 'unable to sleep, had impaired concentration, was not coping domestically and constantly worrying about her responsibilities, afraid to go out of doors, and wondering if the drugs she had been prescribed were harmful to her'. He also commented that she 'was worried that some form of accident or illness will happen to her children, and yet cannot face up to her responsibilities as a mother'. On examination she was noted to be 'morbid, anxious and depressed in mood and to have long-standing feelings of insecurity'. She was admitted to hospital and her drug treatment changed to a different antidepressant (nortriptyline). Three weeks later she was reported to be 'bright and cheerful' but when she went home again she was more tense and anxious. When asked by her new doctor about the reason for her improvement she warmly declared that it was nothing to do with the tablets. She had been allowed to sit around with other patients (mostly women) in groups and they had swapped each other's symptoms at length. This reassured her that there were many other fellow sufferers, and the absence of any responsibilities in hospital apart from taking her turn in the 'washing-up rota' also helped what she called her 'rest cure'. Her diagnosis on discharge was 'depressive neurosis in an inadequate personality' and afterwards she continued to attend as a day-patient. Throughout this period she continued to take antidepressants in the form of nortriptyline (75 mg daily) and tranquillisers in the form of diazepam (10 mg daily).

She improved a little but realised that no new initiatives were planned and soon asked to return to the care of her general practitioner. When her symptoms became worse again nine months later she asked to be re-referred as even if the day-hospital team could not do much more it was reassuring to know that they understood her feelings. This time it was noted that her anxiety symptoms were by far the most prominent and she had no consistent feelings of depression. She found that anxiety about every real or imagined stress dominated her life. As she found it difficult to convey how unpleasant these feelings were she wrote a leter to one of the doctors at the day hospital. This was written in the early hours one morning when her usual insomnia at least allowed her time to collect her thoughts and feelings together.

> I feel frightened and panicky all the time; my head seems to drive me mad, I can't think of anything but my nerves. No matter how hard I try to forget them I can't and it just drives me into a state. I am frightened of everything; ridiculous things like going to bed at night because I know I am going to lie there and not go to sleep. Of course I don't sleep because worrying about it makes me feel more tensed up forcing myself to think about going to sleep. When I try to relax I just see myself from outside trying to relax and it just seems silly. Then as I lie in bed not sleeping I forget about not going to sleep and start to worry about the morning because I am afraid of the day ahead. I just get frightened of every single thing. I am afraid to go out and be with people because I get myself into a panic by thinking that they are

bound to say something that will upset me because I am terribly morbid-minded. I get upset over the slightest thing. If either of my children seem ill in some way or another I get panicky because I always think the worst. I am so frightened of anything happening to them, my husband or me as well.

I am frightened of taking these nerve tablets and sleeping tablets [this letter was written long before official concern about tranquilliser dependence] and of course that makes me even more frightened because I am afraid I will never be able to do without them. My body aches all over and so I can't do all my chores. The next day I get so tired and tensed up. Then I worry about not being able to cope with all the things there are to do in the day, so this gets me into a state. If only I could relax and not worry, I know I could cope. But now I am so tired and exhausted everything I have to do is like climbing a mountain and never getting to the top. I keep crying all the time because I feel absolutely rotten. I got into a real state in bed last night, I thought I was going to die or that you would put me away when you heard about how I was.

This letter was written at a time when superficially there were no particular stresses in the household. Mrs Green was happily married to a husband who was understanding and helpful although, being of a placid nature, he could never understand why his wife became so anxious. Their two children posed no obvious problems in their care and her responsibilities at home were in no way abnormal.

A year later she developed a series of checking rituals lasting half an hour before going to bed at night. This checking involved going around the house looking at each power point and electrical device, and examining all the radiators in the house in turn in case one or more of them might be dripping. When prevented from carrying out these rituals, she could not sleep at night because she could not prevent herself from thinking about the terrible consequences of a leaking or burst radiator. A diagnosis of obsessional (compulsive) neurosis was made and she was referred to a clinical psychologist for treatment. Psychological assessment suggested that 'the present obsessional disorder occurs in the context of long-standing neurotic adjustment in which somewhat hysterical failure to come to terms with adult difficulties is evident'. She was treated by a behavioural approach – response prevention – but made little improvement. Her dosage of diazepam was increased slowly to 10 mg twice daily.

Attempts were made to reduce her medication without success and soon she increased her diazepam further to 30 mg daily. By this time she had repeated episodes of panic associated with hyperventilation and had become preoccupied with the idea that she had a serious illness. At times her panicky feeling led to attacks of vomiting and because of these she was afraid to travel out of doors. Soon she was reluctant to go into any public place for fear of humiliating herself by vomiting uncontrollably.

She was again recommended to attend the hospital as a day-patient. There she joined a group of similar people, all with phobias of different kinds, and was treated by specific behavioural and psychological treatments, including desensitisation and assertive training. Although she made some progress in overcoming her worst fears her tension and panic increased and at times she felt suicidal. However, her predominant feelings were of being trapped, and a fear of both life and death; she was quite unable to cope with any level of responsibility.

She then received a course of individual psychotherapy but found this so distressing that she had to end it after two months. By this time she had developed obsessional thinking in an attempt to ward off imaginary dangers and this reduced her effectiveness still further. She felt compelled to think about each of her family in turn to ensure that they remained well and healthy. She continued to take diazepam in a dose of 20 mg daily and did not feel able to reduce this. The only time she improved was when she went on a short holiday with her family and was completely relieved of any responsibility. She sat all day doing nothing but felt free of tension for the first time for many years. As soon as she returned from holiday her old feelings returned and at different times her fears and obsessions intruded to a greater degree.

How should we classify the disorder shown by this patient? This question, and similar ones concerning conditions that are less complicated than that of Mrs Green, are the subject of this book and the answers are not easy ones. Mrs Green is not a freak, and her account is by no means exceptional. Most professionals concerned with the care of the mentally ill will be reminded of similar patients in their own practice after reading about her. The adjective 'neurotic' is bound to come to mind in describing at least some of the feature shown by her condition, and using current classifications she would undoubtedly have to be placed in one of the categories of neurotic disorder. Unfortunately 'neurotic' is one of those adaptable words that can describe several concepts simultaneously. It covers at least three different concepts: (1) symptoms such as those of anxiety, hypochondriasis, depression and phobias, (2) impairment of function in coping with day-to-day problems (neurotic maladjustment) and (3) an underlying disturbance of character or personality. This accounts for the pejorative use of the adjective, as 'neurotic' carries with it the notion that the symptoms that are causing concern are not really serious, that the patient complains too much about them and that with an effort of will they could be overcome.

These views about neurosis are not recent ones but before the twentieth century the word was used infrequently. In common language 'nervous' covered most of the features included under the heading of neurosis, and neurotic disorder usually carried the same, somewhat negative, connotations. The adjective also included the idea of a long-lasting, underlying personality disturbance. Thus when Mrs Bennett in Jane Austen's *Pride and Prejudice* complains to her husband, 'You have no compassion on my poor nerves', he replies warmly, 'You mistake me, my dear. I have a high respect for your nerves. They are my old friends. I have heard you mention them with consideration these twenty years at least.' Poor Mrs Bennett would doubtless be ascribed one of the labels of neurotic disorder were she to present to a psychiatrist today, although whether this label would describe Mrs Bennett's problems more accurately than Jane Austen is doubtful.

Although this book is concerned with the classification of neurosis it will inevitably cover some of the issues that make 'neurotic' a term of description, criticism and irritation. Unfortunately all these three words can apply to the classification process itself. In current descriptive terminology the condition of the woman with the long-standing problem outlined above satisfies the current diagnostic criteria for generalised anxiety disorder, depressive episode, dysthymic disorder, panic disorder, agoraphobia with panic disorder, obsessive–compulsive neurosis, hypochondriacal syndrome, and at least two personality disorders (obsessive–compulsive and avoidant) at different times. This panoply of names only poses further questions? Does Mrs Green's diagnosis change in an understandable and predictable way or is it unpredictable? Has she a primary disorder and secondary complications or are all her symptoms part of one disorder? Should one disorder take precedence in description even if others are acknowledged as well?

Many clinicians, of whom psychotherapists are perhaps the most prominent, regard the exercise of diagnosis in neurotic disorder as valueless, but there are good reasons for developing a classification. Although attempting to classify Mrs Green's problems may appear to be a labour of Sisyphus, many other neurotic disorders are easier to classify and fit more easily into current schemata. As well as giving order to mental illness classification needs to be useful to the clinician. For a classification to be successful it should not only identify common features but indicate how the disorder is caused, give guidance on treatment and predict the outcome. These requirements are exacting, but necessary. We demand them of classification for other medical disorders and refinement continues until these goals are achieved. If we do not have the same standards in classifying neurotic disorder there will continue to be a significant band of therapists who abandon the idea of diagnosis altogether as an esoteric and largely academic exercise which interferes with, rather than helps, understanding of patients' problems. This view has some substance and when clinicians are presented with problems like those of Mrs Green it is understandable that they become frustrated by the deficiencies of their diagnostic training and return to using personal and idiosyncratic systems that at least appear to have some practical value. But they should not despair altogether and neither should Mrs Green. The easy problems are now being classified well and there are solutions on the horizon for the difficult ones.

# CHAPTER 1

# Neurosis and the International Classification of Diseases

The International Classification of Diseases (ICD) is the only world-wide classification of mental disorders and therefore has a major influence on psychiatric thought and practice. The World Health Organization is responsible for regular revisions of the classification and these are published with a numbered suffix at the time of publication. Nine revisions of ICD have taken place since the first classification appeared in 1900. ICD-9 was published in 1978 and the tenth revision is undergoing field trials at present and is likely to be published in 1990. However, the proposed tenth revision has already been produced in draft form and is currently undergoing field trials. Extracts from the draft revision are reproduced with special permission of the World Health Organization. There is no guarantee that the draft revision will persist unchanged into the final version of ICD-10 but the main diagnostic categories are unlikely to change.

The neurotic disorders are placed in a separate group in the classification together with stress-related and somatoform disorders. As stress-related and somatoform disorders have such close relationships with the other neurotic disorders they are included within the group in this book. In addition there is some overlap between the neurotic disorders and mood (affective) disorders and with that other section of ICD entitled 'physiological dysfunction associated with mental and behavioural factors'. All forms of depression are placed in the section on mood disorders and this

Table 1.1 Proposed classification of neurotic disorders and associated conditions in the draft version of ICD-10

| Individual Diagnosis | Subclassification |
| --- | --- |
| Phobic disorder | Agoraphobia<br>Social phobia<br>Isolated phobia |
| Other anxiety disorder | Panic<br>Generalized<br>Mixed anxiety–depressive |
| Obsessive–compulsive disorder | Obsessional thoughts and ruminations<br>Obsessional rituals (compulsive acts)<br>Mixed obsessional thoughts and acts |
| Dissociative disorder<br>  memory, awareness and identity | Psychogenic amnesia<br>Psychogenic fugue<br>Psychogenic stupor<br>Trance and possession states |
|   movement and sensation | Psychogenic disorders of voluntary movement<br>Psychogenic convulsions<br>Psychogenic anaesthesia and sensory loss<br>Other dissociative disorder<br>Unspecified dissociative or conversion disorder |
| Somatoform disorder | Somatization disorder<br>Undifferentiated somatization disorder<br>Hypochondriacal syndrome<br>Psychogenic autonomic dysfunction<br>Pain syndrome without specific organic cause<br>Other psychogenic disorder of sensation, function and behaviour |
| Other neurotic disorder | Neurasthenia (fatigue syndrome)<br>Depersonalization–derealization syndrome |
| Unspecified neurotic, stress-related or somatoform disorder | |

| Main Diagnostic Grouping | Individual Diagnosis | Subclassification | Reason for Inclusion in Relationship to a Neurotic Disorder |
|---|---|---|---|
| Mood (affective disorder) | Depressive episode Recurrent depressive disorders Persistent affective states | Mild depressive episode Recurrent mild depressive disorder Dysthymia | Formerly included in neurotic disorder as depressive neurosis in previous revisions of ICD |
| Physiological dysfunction associated with mental or behavioural factors | Eating disorders | Obesity associated with other psychological disturbance Vomiting associated with other psychological disturbance | Associated psychological disturbance, often a neurotic disorder |
| | Sleep and arousal disorders | Insomnia Hypersomnia Disorders of the sleep–wake cycle Sleep terrors Nightmares (dream anxiety) | Frequent symptoms in anxiety disorder |
| | Sexual dysfunctions | Lack or loss of sexual desire | Commonly associated with other neurotic symptoms |
| | Psychological distress related to the menstrual cycle | Premenstrual tension syndrome | |
| Abnormalities of adult personality and behaviour | Personality disorders | Anankastic Anxious Dependent | Frequently coexist with neurotic disorder |

includes the milder forms formerly classified as depressive neu rosis. The diagnoses now covered by this group are shown togethe with the other neurotic disorders in Table 1.1. Among the disorder of physiological dysfunction are those of sleep, and several of thes overlap with the neuroses. Some of the sexual dysfunctions shoul also be considered under this heading (Table 1.2).

Unlike previous editions of ICD, the draft version of ICD-1 includes diagnostic guidelines. These list general criteria for inclu sion in a particular diagnostic category but fall somewhat short c the operational criteria that are intrinsic to the American classifica tions. The diagnostic guidelines in ICD-10 'indicate the number an balance of symptoms usually required before a confident diagnosi can be made, but they are phrased so that a degree of flexibility i retained in the diagnostic decision' (World Health Organizatior 1988).

In the earlier revisions of ICD neurosis and psychosis are sepa rated clearly and depressive neurosis is one of the main categories i the neurotic group. The others are anxiety; hysterical, phobic obsessional, and hypochondriacal neuroses; depersonalization an neurasthenia. The major advantage of ICD-10 over previou revisions of ICD when describing depressive disorders is that a patients with a primary complaint of depression are covered in th mood disorder section of ICD-10. In previous versions depressio appears in as many colours as the chameleon throughout th classification. For example, in ICD-9 depression appears as primary disorder in a section on affective psychoses (ICD no. 296) other non-organic psychoses (298), neurotic disorders (300), person ality disorders (as affective personality disorder) (301) and, for th unusual case which cannot satisfy any of the above categories, ther is a separate, all-embracing category of 'depressive disorder no elsewhere classified' (311) (World Health Organization, 1978) ICD-10 is certainly an improvement on this.

## EATING DISORDERS

There are several diagnoses in the general category of physiologica dysfunction that are closely linked to neurotic disorders. Among th eating disorders anorexia nervosa and bulimia nervosa are suffi ciently distinct to be excluded from consideration but obesity an vomiting associated with other psychological disturbance are botl often found in the presence of neuroses and frequently a funda mental part of them. In the draft of ICD-10 obesity is said t sometimes follow distressing events such as bereavements, oper itions and childbirth. This 'reactive obesity' can easily be viewed as an unusual type of stress and adjustment disorder and is unlikely to be a sole symptom, although in the long term it may be the only legacy of the event. Obesity itself can also provoke emotional reactions and 'cause the patient to feel sensitive about his or her appearance and give rise to a lack of confidence in personal relationships'. Dieting may also lead to anxiety, depression and irritability and thus can be included in this category. The general finding in epidemiological studies that fat people are jolly (Crisp and McGuiness, 1976) has many unfortunate exceptions. The third suggested category in this section is obesity occurring as a consequence of long-term consumption of antidepressant or neuroleptic drugs. This is an important and serious problem of long-term therapy but clearly is a separate disorder independent of neurosis (except in those patients taking long-term antidepressants for neurotic disturbance).

Vomiting as a repeated problem is said in the draft to occur in dissociative disorders, hypochondriasis and pregnancy. It may also be a phobic disorder although it is not for some reason included in the list of isolated phobias. Again the association with neurotic disorder is strong and demands discussion.

## SLEEP AND AROUSAL DISORDERS

Sleep, Shakespeare's 'chief nourisher in life's feast', is one of the first functions to suffer in the neuroses and some may regard it as odd that insomnia is allowed separate diagnostic status in ICD-10. However, sleep disorders, including insomnia, have long been offered a separate diagnostic coding (307.4 in ICD-9) when 'a more precise medical or psychiatric diagnosis cannot be made'. In ICD-10 the guidelines make it clear that the diagnosis of insomnia should only be made when 'unsatisfactory quality and/or quality of sleep' is the only complaint or at least the primary one in the patients' perception. However, as anxiety, depression, obsessional and hypochondriacal symptoms can all occur in insomnia (and be separately coded in ICD-10) it is necessary to include insomnia as a condition that is more usually associated with neurotic symptomatology than any other group of disorders.

Hypersomnia, defined as 'excessive daytime sleepiness and sleep attacks, or prolonged transition to the fully aroused state on wakening (sleep drunkenness)', is much less commonly associated with neurotic disorder. It can only be diagnosed in the absence of narcolepsy or sleep apnoea; the rare Kleine Levin syndrome, where hypersomnia is associated with excessive eating (megaphagia) and weight gain; or of cerebral organic disorders such as encephalitis

Disorders of the sleep–wake cycle, formerly termed 'inversion of sleep rhythm', are also described in some detail in ICD-10. They are defined somewhat clumsily as 'a lack of synchrony between the patient's sleep–wake schedule and the desired sleep–wake schedules for his/her environment resulting in a complaint of either insomnia or hypersomnia'. This diagnosis owes much to interest in biorhythms, the notion that certain basic drives have an endogenous component that resists our attempt to force them into patterns of our choosing. Expressions such as 'intrinsic malfunction of the individual's circadian oscillator' indicate the impact of this biological thinking. These disorders are only occasionally associated with neurotic symptomatology but are included for completeness

Sleep terrors (*pavor nocturnus*) are included as an associated condition because their major characteristics, panic and intense autonomic and somatic symptoms, are similar to those of daytime panic. This disorder has been regarded as a significant and symbolic component of neurotic symptomatology since Freud's early writings (Freud, 1895a, but in ICD-10 is seen in diagnostic terms as a more extreme variant of sleep walking. Epilepsy needs to be excluded before making the diagnosis. Nightmares are also given separate diagnostic status and are differentiated from sleep terrors by their high incidence in the last hour of sleep, immediate recall of the dream which has a common theme of threat, and a greater degree of psychopathology, said in ICD-10 usually to be that of a personality disorder. Sleep terrors generally occur in the first few hours of sleep and are seldom recalled. Dreams and nightmares take place during rapid eye movements (REM) sleep and are suppressed by several drugs, often completely by barbiturates, and when these drugs are stopped there is a greater amount of REM sleep (rebound) and consequently a greater risk of nightmares. Although nightmares occurring in this situation are iatrogenic they can still satisfy the diagnostic criteria for nightmares. Many patients affected in this way have an additional neurotic diagnosis which was responsible for the original prescription of the offending drug.

## SEXUAL DYSFUNCTIONS

Sex has a special place in neurosis and for some is the most prominent feature. The diagnostic range in ICD-10 includes lack or loss of sexual desire, lack of sexual enjoyment, failure of genital response, orgasmic dysfunction, premature ejaculation, vag inismus (vaginal occlusion due to pelvic muscle spasm) and dyspareunia (painful intercourse). Psychological distress related to the menstrual cycle (particularly premenstrual tension syndrome) also makes its appearance in ICD-10 for the first time. This is defined as a cyclical condition with handicapping symptoms which have 'a consistent and predictable relationship to menstruation'. Only one symptom from the following list is needed to satisfy the diagnosis if its relationship to menstruation is established: irritability, depression, bloating and weight gain, breast tenderness, tension, aches and pains, difficulty in concentration and physiological change (appetite and sleep disturbance). The list of symptoms is so catholic and unrestricted that virtually all who complain of symptoms related to menstruation will satisfy the diagnosis. The diagnosis is likely to be regarded as sexist in many quarters.

## PERSONALITY DISORDERS

It has long been known that there is an association between neurosis and personality disorder. Indeed, the association has sometimes been taken so much for granted that psychiatric textbooks frequently include personality disorders in the same section as neurotic ones, the implication being that they merge imperceptibly with one another. This association has developed from psychoanalytical writings in the first 50 years of this century. Freud (1908) and Alexander (1930) used the words 'neurotic character' and 'character neurosis' to describe a group of patients within the spectrum of neurosis. Those with 'pure' neuroses developed symptoms that were out of keeping with their normal function and regarded as quite alien. Others had similar symptoms over a much longer period and regarded them as intrinsic parts of their nature, whether or not they were unpleasant. Alexander (1930) coined the term 'ego-dystonic' to describe the first group and 'ego-syntonic' to describe the second group of character neuroses. Not surprisingly, the ego-syntonic group were much more difficult to treat with psychotherapy.

The concept of personality disorder was already well established before the psychoanalytical era but, particularly through the influence of Koch (1891), has been imbued with the notion of degeneracy and asocial or antisocial behaviour. The recognition that the milder degrees of psychiatric symptomatology overlapped to some extent with abnormal personality was a new and important finding. It established that the concept of personality disorder as a single entity was unlikely to be useful and led indirectly to the main categories of

Table 1.3  Comparison of current classifications of personality disorder

| Code | DSM-III-R | ICD-10 | Code |
|---|---|---|---|
| 301.00 | Paranoid – interpretation of people's actions as deliberately demeaning or threatening | Paranoid – excessive sensitivity, suspiciousness, preoccupation with conspiratorial explanation of events, with a persistent tendency to self-reference | F 60.0 |
| 301.20 | Schizoid – indifference to social relationships and restricted range of emotional experience and expression | Schizoid – emotional coldness, detachment, lack of interest in other people, eccentricity and introspective fantasy | F 60.1 |
| 301.22 | Schizotypal – deficit in interpersonal relatedness with peculiarities of ideation, appearance and behaviour | No equivalent | |
| 301.40 | Obsessive–Compulsive – pervasive perfectionism and inflexibility | Anankastic – indecisiveness, doubt, excessive caution, pedantry, rigidity and need to plan in immaculate detail | F 60.5 |
| 301.50 | Histrionic – excessive emotionality and attention-seeking | Histrionic – self-dramatisation, shallow mood, egocentricity and craving for excitement with persistent manipulative behaviour | F 60.4 |
| 301.60 | Dependent – persistent dependent and submissive behaviour | Dependent – failure to take responsibility for actions, with subordination of personal needs to those of others, excessive dependence with need for constant reassurance and feelings of helplessness when a close relationship ends | F 60.7 |

| | | | |
|---|---|---|---|
| 301.70 | Antisocial – evidence of repeated conduct disorder before the age of 15 | Dyssocial – callous unconcern for others, with irresponsibility, irritability and aggression, and incapacity to maintain enduring relationships | F 60.2 |
| 301.81 | Narcissistic – pervasive grandiosity, lack of empathy, and hypersensitivity to the evaluation of others | No equivalent | |
| 301.82 | Avoidant – pervasive social discomfort, fear of negative evaluation and timidity | Anxious – persistent tension, self-consciousness, exaggeration of risks and dangers, hypersensitivity to rejection, and restricted lifestyle because of insecurity | F 60.6 |
| 301.83 | Borderline – pervasive instability of mood, and self-image | Impulsive – inability to control anger, to plan ahead, or to think before acts, with unpredictable mood and quarrelsome behaviour | F 60.30* |
| | | Borderline – unclear self-image, involvement in intense and unstable relationships | F 60.31* |
| 301.84 | Passive–Aggressive – pervasive passive resistance to demands for adequate social and occupational performance | No equivalent | |

* Included under heading of emotionally unstable personality disorder.

abnormal personality in successive classifications of ICD. Nevertheless, it is unfortunate that personality disorder has been linked so strongly with neurosis. Studies of the co-occurrence of personality disorder and different psychiatric diagnoses have demonstrated that whereas about 38% of patients with neurotic disorder have associated personality disturbance the rates are higher for adjustment disorders (50%), schizophrenia (55%) and alcohol dependence (69%) (Tyrer *et al.*, 1988a).

The categorisation of personality disorder in the revised third edition of the *Diagnostic and Statistical Manual of Mental Disorders* (DSM-III-R; American Psychiatric Association, 1987) and in the draft version of ICD-10 is shown in Table 1.3. The differences are relatively small and are mainly shown by the inclusion of borderline, narcissistic and passive–aggressive personality disorders in DSM-III-R (and DSM-III; American Psychiatric Association, 1980). However, in the latest revision of ICD-10, borderline personality disorder is included as one of the subdivisions of emotionally unstable personality disorder. There are two additional diagnoses in DSM-III-R which are not yet accepted as formal diagnoses: the sadistic and self-defeating personality disorders. Another new category, anxious personality disorder, has been introduced in ICD-10 in response to the inclusion of avoidant personality disorder in DSM-III-R. This describes the avoiding patterns of behaviour by those who are commonly anxious but as it is the behaviour rather than the mood state that we regard as important it could be more accurately described as avoidant personality disorder, and indeed the word 'avoidant' accompanies this category.

A constant problem of classification in psychiatry is the dividing line between mental state and personality disorders and this will recur in subsequent chapters. Neurotic disorders are more commonly associated with anankastic, dependent and histrionic personality types than with the other categories and dependence is perhaps their most consistent feature (Tyrer *et al.*, 1986). Until recently there has been a somewhat sterile debate over whether an individual patient suffers from a personality disorder or a neurosis. It is now realised that personality status constitutes a separate axis of classification and the more correct question is: has this patient with a neurotic condition an associated personality abnormality or disorder? The co-occurrence of any personality abnormality does not change the diagnosis of neurosis; it just adds to it.

The most common difficulty in deciding whether or not a neurosis is associated with personality disorder is when chronic conditions are considered. It has been known for over 20 years that the personality characteristics of patients with mental illness can alter temporarily during the course of illness (Coppen and Metcalfe, 1965) and so it is important to assess personality status in the absence of other mental illness. However, in the case of a chronic disorder it is difficult to find any significant period of time that is free of illness. In these circumstances the diagnosis of personality disorder cannot really be made because the satisfactory information is lacking, yet at the same time it could be argued that as the handicaps produced are typical of that person's behaviour and functioning the condition could be included in the personality domain.

An important change has taken place in the classification of neurosis in the last ten years. The earlier editions of ICD made a broad separation between the psychoses and the neuroses together with personality disorders and associated conditions. In ICD-9 the psychoses are defined as disorders 'in which impairment of mental function has developed to a degree that interferes grossly with insight, ability to meet some ordinary demands of life or to maintain adequate contact with reality' (World Health Organization, 1978). Neurotic disorders are the obverse of this coin of classification, being 'disorders without any demonstrable organic basis in which the patient may have considerable insight and have unimpaired reality testing, in that he does not confuse his morbid subjective experiences and fantasies with external reality'. Thus the psychotic patient is very ill and does not realise it whereas the neurotic patient is less ill and realises it almost too well.

This classification, based on the rather nebulous tenets of insight and reality testing, is not particularly satisfactory. This was realised to some extent in ICD-8 and ICD-9, retained because of historical tradition, but in ICD-10 has been abandoned. Thus although most of the established neurotic disorders appear together in the classification, because of the generally agnostic approach that allows diagnosis to be 'simply a set of symptoms that have been agreed by a large number of advisers and consultants from many different countries, as a reasonable basis for defining "typical" disorders', they can appear in different conditions throughout the classification. In view of this different approach it is perhaps surprising that the concept of neurotic disorders has not been abandoned altogether. The retaining link appears to be aetiology, although this is frowned upon in a classification that is primarily concerned with the formal description of symptoms and behaviour. This is acknowledged apologetically in the introduction to the ICD-10 section on neurotic, stress-related and somatoform disorders, which are included together 'because of their historical association with the concept of neurosis, and the association of a substantial (though not exactly known) proportion of these disorders with psychological causation'. When the old ties are difficult to break they have greater meaning.

CHAPTER 2

# Neurosis: The American Perspective

In recent years the term 'neurosis' has been disparaged in many quarters, but particularly in the United States where the abandonment of the word as a diagnostic term has been a *cause célèbre*. This is because the debate pitted the two great schools of psychiatry, the psychodynamic and the phenomenological, against each other and had far more implications than the mere use of the word.

The controversy was stimulated by the development of DSM-III. Until DSM-III the American classification had been very similar to ICD, although there were some important differences. However, the pressure for a satisfactory classification that was fundamentally atheoretical and reliable was strong and was particularly needed by research workers in psychiatry. The DSM-III Task Force, under the energetic chairmanship of Robert Spitzer, set about making major revisions and introduced operational criteria to improve the reliability of the individual categories. This was bound to create controversy, both political and scientific, and the intensity of the debate created by the initial proposals of the Task Force has only recently become generally known in published papers. One of the great merits of American society is its openness: there is no field in which controversy remains secret for long and its general discussion is extremely valuable to those involved in evaluating changes. Similar dissemination of debate could be of value in more secretive European countries.

Because DSM-III set out deliberately to adopt an empirical stance towards diagnosis there was bound to be controversy over neuroses. Even when the second revision of DSM was being prepared an attempt was made to avoid adopting a doctrinaire position about the character or cause of conditions for which no satisfactory knowledge was available (Gruenberg, 1969). At that time, however, the psychoanalytic movement in the United States was extremely strong and the changes recommended by the DSM-II Task Force were not all realised.

The DSM-III Task Force was made of sterner stuff and had more weapons at its disposal. 'Neurosis' as a term had to be eliminated from the classification because 'as a unifying theme for explicating and co-ordinating diverse syndromes it had outlived its usefulness both as a nomenclature designation and as a classificatory principle (Millon, 1983).

What happened next has been discussed fully by Bayer and Spitzer (1985). They described the debate as one between a group who were 'atheoretical with regard to what they believed were unproved aetiological assumptions, and who therefore pressed for a criteria-based classification that would be reliable and could provide the basis for testable hypotheses' and a second group 'who argued that decades of experience with the clinically complex issues involved in psychotherapeutic work with patients had established the validity of the psychodynamic perspective'. The DSM-III Task Force dominated the first group and were determined to do without neurosis in their new classification. The term implied intrapsychic conflict as a cause of neurotic symptoms, but the group could find no evidence that this type of conflict was involved in all those cases labelled as neurotic.

The psychodynamic school were unhappy that the new classification was based only on 'shared phenomenological characteristics and ignored the role of the unconscious and psychodynamic conflict. There was concern that the new classification would hinder rather than help the treatment of patients in psychoanalysis, summarised by Schimel as a 'retreat from a psychiatry of people'. The psychodynamic critics focused their attack on the restrictive nature of the new classification, using terms such as 'linguistic and conceptual sterility' and 'rigid exclusionism' in criticising the limits of description that had been set (Burgh, cited by Bayer and Spitzer 1985). Attempts were made to include psychodynamic data in the description of each of the neurotic disorders since 'psychiatric diagnoses made only on the basis of science and symptoms, without a positive psychodynamically informed, coherent understanding of why the patient has developed the symptom at this time is second rate diagnosis' (Rockland, cited by Bayer and Spitzer, 1985).

The reason why the word 'neurosis' became so emotionally charged is that it reflected the dynamic implications of diagnosis in a way that 'neurotic disorder' did not. Like most debates that are carried out between equally powerful groups, there was no obvious victor or vanquished at the end of the argument. The term 'neurosis' was eliminated as such in the classification, but the inclusion of 'anxiety neurosis' and 'neurotic depression' in parentheses represented a victory of sorts for the dynamic school. The replacement of 'neurosis' with 'neurotic disorder' could hardly be regarded as a major classificatory change. As an editorial in the *Lancet* neatly put it after reviewing DSM–III: 'neurosis is not dead, it has merely retreated in disorder' (*Lancet*, 1982).

Viewed from the other side of the Atlantic the angry debates about classification in the United States sometimes led to patronising amusement. It was easy to see the Americans as uncritical enthusiasts who were governed by fad and fashion rather than reflection and so accounted for the major swings in American psychiatry. Thus the wholehearted embrace of psychoanalysis by America in the first half of this century has been seen as being replaced by a love affair with scientific psychiatry in which every statement has to rely on objective criteria that have been developed through testable hypotheses. Such lofty superiority is unjustified and American psychiatry, through its enthusiasm, openness, and organisation in the form of many task forces, has generated changes that have affected the subject internationally. These will become apparent during the reading of this book and show particularly strongly in the adoption of many American developments in the new revision of ICD (ICD-10). The writer accepts the validity of many of these changes, but differs in retaining the word 'neurosis' throughout this book. This is purely for reasons of economy; there is no point in using two words when one conveys exactly the same information. Those who wish to translate 'neurosis' into 'neurotic disorder' may do so, although I hope that others can retain their peace of mind in tolerating the original.

To keep to the spirit of intent in DSM-III and DSM-III-R there are no tables of DSM 'neuroses' in this chapter. In any case, their close similarity and overlap with the proposed ICD-10 classification would only duplicate the tables in the previous chapter. Many American readers would be unhappy about all these disorders being brought together under the collective umbrella of neurosis. Aubrey Lewis (1975) referred to 'hysteria' as a tough old word that would tend to outlive its obituarists. 'Neurosis' is even tougher: it predates psychoanalysis by 150 years and, although Freud and his followers added a great number of aetiological implications to the term, they did not alter its basic description. It will not be discarded easily and it has sufficient unifying characteristics for its advocates to be confident in its defence.

# CHAPTER 3

# Panic and Generalized Anxiety Disorder

Before 1980 the classification of anxiety disorders appeared to be straightforward and, perhaps, somewhat boring. Anxiety was classified as a single disorder usually under the heading of 'anxiety neurosis', 'anxiety state' or 'anxiety reaction'. The primary symptom was that of anxiety in both its psychological and bodily forms and in severe cases the symptoms could be described as panic. The diagnosis of anxiety neurosis appeared to be a fairly stable one and had survived since Sigmund Freud first described the condition as a separate diagnostic syndrome in 1895a.

Freud, like all good nosologists, felt that when certain symptoms grouped together they could be given a common identity, and so he suggested that a syndrome could be detached from the concept of neurasthenia that was prevalent in his time. Although Freud is given credit for introducing the diagnosis he acknowledges in his paper that the condition has been described earlier by Hecker (1893) in the German literature. However, Freud's description is the only one that is remembered. This is not surprising as Freud had a felicity of style that made all his contributions eminently readable.

Freud described ten common features in anxiety neurosis: general irritability, anxious expectation, free-floating anxiousness, anxiety attacks, nocturnal terror, vertigo, the development of phobias, gastrointestinal disturbance, paraesthesias and a tendency towards chronicity. These features can hardly be improved upon as a description of the predominant features of pathological anxiety.

17

Freud's description of anxiety attacks is also apposite in view of the recent classification of panic disorder as a separate diagnostic entity. He points out that anxiousness 'can suddenly break through into consciousness without being aroused by a train of ideas, and thus provoke an anxiety attack. An anxiety attack of this sort may consist of the feeling of anxiety alone, without any associated idea, or accompanied by the interpretation that is nearest to hand, such as ideas of the extinction of life, or of a stroke, or of a threat of madness; or else some kind of paraesthesia (similar to the hysterical aura) may be combined with the feeling of anxiety, or, finally, the feeling of anxiety may have linked to it a disturbance of one or more of the bodily functions – such as respiration, heart action, vasomotor innervation, or glandular activity' (Freud, 1895). This account emphasises the three characteristic features of panic attacks: their unpredictability, their lack of association with any known stimulus, and their presentation as a fear of going mad or dying mixed together with various bodily symptoms. Because these symptoms are commonly found together subsequent attempts at classifying anxiety make very few changes to the Freudian prototype. Freud himself made another important contribution in his 1926 paper when he distinguished between 'normal anxiety' as 'anxiety about a known danger' and 'neurotic anxiety' as 'anxiety about a danger that has yet to be discovered'. This absence of any relationship between the anxiety and an understandable threat is one of the key features that makes pathological anxiety a psychiatric disorder.

Freud would probably have found little to take exception to in the ICD-9 description of anxiety states, which is merely a précis of his own papers:

> Various combinations of physical and mental manifestations of anxiety, not attributable to real danger and occurring either in attacks or as a persisting state. The anxiety is usually diffuse and may extend to panic. Other neurotic features such as obsessional or hysterical symptoms may be present, but do not dominate the clinical picture. (World Health Organization, 1978)

## COMPARISON BETWEEN GENERALIZED ANXIETY AND PANIC DISORDER

The diagnosis of panic disorder is one of the newest additions to psychiatric classification. It was first identified as a diagnostic entity in DSM-III, has been refined further in DSM-III-R and is also a diagnosis in ICD-10. Anxiety disorders are now separated into panic disorder and generalized anxiety disorder and the reasoning behind this important change needs full discussion.

The word 'panic' has an interesting derivation. The cloven-footed Greek god, Pan, with the upper torso and face of a man but body of a beast, had an impish sense of humour and loved playing practical jokes on man. Travellers in the Greek region of Arcadia used to be fairly frightened when passing through the forests of the region, which were home to many wild animals. Pan used to delight in jumping out of the undergrowth in front of them, only to disappear again equally quickly. The acute anxiety and terror felt by the travellers were labelled 'panic' after their originator. However, this description differs from that now commonly used to describe panics, most of which occur in the absence of any identifiable stimulus. One of the best descriptions of these apparently spontaneous attacks of panic was given by Freud in his 1895 paper when he argued for the existence of anxiety neurosis as a separate diagnostic entity. He emphasised that the emotion of anxiety could occur suddenly, without warning and without being called forth by any train of thought. These anxiety attacks were often associated with fears of death, physical or mental catastrophes, and associated with marked bodily symptoms (p. 18). Interestingly enough, although Freud included these panic attacks in his argument for the separation of anxiety neurosis as a diagnosis (i.e. for including what is now called generalized anxiety disorder and panic disorder in one group) he did not argue for panic as a specific diagnosis. Yet his description, reinforced by more recent authorities, particularly Donald Klein in New York, has become the cornerstone of the new diagnosis for panic disorder.

The reason why panic was detached from the superstructure of anxiety neurosis and set apart to form the basis of a new edifice was, like many changes in classification, a consequence of treatment. In two early papers (Klein and Fink, 1962; Klein, 1964) the beneficial effect of imipramine in relieving the symptom of panic was described. It was also noted that this effect was independent of background generalised anxiety. Patients stopped running to the nursing station for help as their panic attacks disappeared but they often remained tense and anxious. However, it was found that the patients whose panic attacks were alleviated did not develop anticipatory anxiety and phobias whereas those whose attacks persisted often did develop these conditions.

Klein concluded that imipramine 'blocked' panic attacks through a specific, and as yet unknown, pharmacological action. He also hypothesised that the spontaneous panic is the 'proximal key causal link that often initiates secondary anticipatory anxiety and the tertiary adaptive dependent phobic behavioural sequence, maintaining them both by an irregular aversive schedule. Such a reversible key symptom is extraordinarily helpful in recognising homogeneous diagnostic sub-groups with predictable benefit to drug treatment' (Klein and Klein, 1989a, p. 136). Klein developed his arguments by postulating that almost all cases of agoraphobia were preceded by spontaneous panic attacks whereas other forms of phobia, including social as well as simple phobias, were not associated with this provoking stimulus. He also provided evidence that separation anxiety in childhood was a common precursor of adult agoraphobia with panic (Gittelman and Klein, 1984).

In order for panic disorder to achieve diagnostic status it was necessary to define its nature clearly and to emphasise the distinctions between it and other forms of anxiety. This was done by postulating a second condition, generalized anxiety disorder, in which there was unfocused anxiety and tension, often with bodily symptoms, but not associated with attacks of panic. A distinction also had to be made between attacks of anxiety occurring only during exposure to an identifiable stimulus, most frequently a phobic one, and attacks that occurred spontaneously in the absence of a stimulus.

The task of defining panic was not difficult and could have been developed from Freud's original description without any additional information. The essential features were: (1) a subjective feeling of panic occurring in the absence of any stimulus (or if occurring in response to a stimulus only happening occasionally and unpredictably), (2) fear of dying, collapsing or losing control and (3) anxiety of such severity as to produce a range of bodily symptoms such as difficulty in breathing, palpitations, tightness in the chest and other bodily accompaniments of anxiety.

The therapeutic implications of this distinction were great. Imipramine, and possibly other antidepressants, might be specific treatments for panic disorder whereas for the more diffuse generalized anxiety other treatments such as relaxation training and sedative drugs such as the benzodiazepines would be more appropriate (Greenblatt and Shader, 1974). This combination of accurate description and therapeutic distinction led to the adoption of panic disorder by the American Psychiatric Association and its inclusion in DSM-III as a diagnosis in its own right.

## Definitions of panic disorder in DSM-III, DSM-III-R and ICD-10

There is reasonably good agreement between the DSM and ICD classifications for panic disorder (Table 3.1) although, as with most of these comparisons, the DSM criteria are more specific. Some minor changes have been made to the DSM-III criteria in the DSM-III-R version. DSM-III only required three panic attacks to occur within a three-week period for the diagnosis, but did not include the additional qualifying requirement of persistent fear of another panic attack. The circumstances of the panic attacks have also been amended. In DSM-III the panic attacks were required to 'occur in circumstances other than life-threatening situations, marked physical exertion or *immediately* before or upon exposure to a situation that *always* causes anxiety or avoidance'. The introduction of the adjective 'almost' into the DSM-III-R description allows panic disorder to be diagnosed in phobic patients who have panic attacks for much, but not all, of the times they are exposed to the situations. However, the exclusion of panic attacks occurring when the person is the focus of others' attention means that many patients with social phobia will not receive the panic disorder diagnosis.

The main difference between the ICD-10 and DSM-III-R descriptions is that most patients with phobic disorders in the ICD-10 classification will not receive a diagnosis of panic. Also, it is not clear whether patients who are persistently anxious but also have attacks of panic could be regarded as having panic anxiety; the diagnostic guidelines suggest that they would not in most cases receive this diagnosis.

## Case histories

### 3.1   *Panic Disorder*

Mrs Gill was a 38-year-old married woman who was referred by her general practitioner because of disabling attacks of anxiety. She had not seen a psychiatrist before, but had had her first attack 20 years previously during difficulties in her first marriage. At that time she had just found out that her husband had been repeatedly unfaithful and, as a consequence, she became anxious and distressed about the future. She developed an acute attack of anxiety without warning one evening when her husband was out. The attack reached a peak within five minutes and lasted for an hour. During the attack she had palpitations, dizziness and sweating, and was convinced that she was going to pass out. She had one other attack six weeks later, but shortly after this she left her husband and the attacks stopped.

She remarried three years later and all went well with this second

Table 3.1  Classification of Panic Disorder in DSM-III, DSM-III-R and ICD-10

| DSM-III | DSM-III-R | ICD-10 (also termed 'episodic paroxysmal anxiety') |
|---|---|---|
| At least three panic attacks (sudden onset of intense apprehension, fear or terror) within a three-week period in circumstances other than during marked physical exertion or in a life threatening situation. The attacks are not precipitated only by exposure to a circumscribed phobic stimulus | At least four panic attacks (discrete periods of intense fear or discomfort) within a four-week period or 'one or more attacks have been followed by a period of at least a month of persistent fear of having another attack'. Attacks must be unexpected, not triggered by situations in which the person was the focus of other's attention | Recurrent attacks of severe anxiety (lasting for minutes only) that are unpredictable and associated with autonomic symptoms, feelings of unreality, and secondary fears of dying, losing control or going mad |
| At least four of the following symptoms during an attack: <br>(i) dyspnoea <br>(ii) palpitations <br>(iii) chest pain or discomfort <br>(iv) choking or smothering sensations | At least four of the following symptoms developed during at least one of the attacks: <br>(i) dyspnoea or smothering sensations <br>(ii) dizziness, unsteadiness or faintness | For definite diagnosis, severe attacks of autonomic anxiety should occur: <br>(i) within a period of about one month <br>(ii) in circumstances where there is no objective danger <br>(iii) not confined to known or |

(v) dizziness
(vi) unreality feelings
(vii) tingling in hands and feet
(viii) hot and cold flushes
(ix) trembling and shaking

(iii) palpitations or tachycardia
(iv) trembling or shaking
(v) sweating
(vi) choking
(vii) nausea or abdominal distress
(viii) depersonalization or derealization
(ix) numbness or tingling sensations
(x) flushes or chills
(xi) chest pain or discomfort
(xii) fear of dying
(xiii) fear of going crazy or doing something uncontrolled

At least four of these symptoms 'developed suddenly and increased in intensity within ten minutes of the beginning of the first symptoms noticed in the attack'

If fewer than four symptoms present the attacks are described as 'limited symptom attacks'

(iv) predictable situations comparative freedom from symptoms between attacks (although mild anticipatory anxiety is common)

Diagnosis to be excluded as a primary one if attacks occur in 'an established phobic situation' or if a phobic disorder or depressive disorder is present

relationship. Her two children of her first marriage continued to live with her and she received regular maintenance payments from her ex-husband. However, in the three months before being referred by her general practitioner her ex-husband had stopped sending money and she was in the midst of taking legal action against him when she had three further panic attacks within the space of 20 days. These were very similar to the ones that she had had originally except that on these occasions she felt even more certain that she would collapse and possibly die. She was already anxious before her first attack because of the problems over maintenance, but her anxiety level increased markedly afterwards because she was so fearful of having more attacks. She had not changed any of her activities since having the attacks apart from avoiding a busy, covered shopping centre over the Christmas period when it was exceptionally busy.

At interview she was apprehensive at first but settled rapidly and showed no observable anxiety by the end of the interview. She had already started to show some improvement on treatment (see p. 38) and so this was continued. One month later the problems over the maintenance of her children had been sorted out with her ex-husband through the courts and she had been able to stop her treatment without any ill effects. She was free of symptoms at follow-up and therefore discharged from further care.

There seems little doubt that this patient would be diagnosed as having panic disorder in DSM-III-R as she had undoubted panic attacks occurring independently of situations and not associated with phobic symptomatology or avoidance. Although she did not have four attacks within a four-week period her concern about having a further attack means that she qualifies for the diagnosis with regard to frequency. She also has five of the symptoms required to make the diagnosis. She probably would also receive a diagnosis of panic disorder using the ICD-10 classification, but as the panic attacks occurred at times when she was more generally anxious there could be doubt as to whether the panic anxiety could be regarded as secondary. However, as the panics were by far the most prominent feature it is likely that the diagnosis would be made. The frequency criterion of 'at least once a week' in ICD-10 is also a little vague. Nevertheless, this patient did have three attacks within a three-week period and would therefore qualify for the diagnosis.

## 3.2 Generalized Anxiety Disorder

Miss Rimms, a 28-year-old clerk, was referred to the outpatient psychiatric clinic by her general practitioner with a request for relaxation training. She had always been somewhat anxious and tense and had developed the habit of overcoming this by eating. Consequently she was considerably overweight and at times felt demoralised and depressed about this. She had been more tense in the three months before referral as her latest boyfriend had broken off his relationship with her.

At interview she was tense and fidgety, talked fast and nervously, had sweaty palms and a rapid pulse of 96 per minute. Her history indicated that her symptoms were of long standing and slightly greater in degree since her boyfriend left. At no time had she had a panic attack and there were no phobic symptoms, and although she had experienced some depressive symptoms they had never lasted for more than a few days at a time. She had difficulty in getting off to sleep and complained of inability to concentrate.

She was treated by a programme of weight reduction, relaxation and anxiety management training. This led to a loss in weight of 15 kg, improvement in her self-esteem and some reduction in her anxiety symptoms. She was pleased at this degree of progress but it was noticeable at further interviews that she was still anxious and tense.

Although there is some overlap between Miss Rimm's problem and adjustment disorder (Chapter 7), and some difficulty in differentiating between her premorbid anxious personality and current symptoms, there is little doubt she would be classified as having generalized anxiety disorder using the latest classifications (Table 3.2).

## ANALYSIS

### Clarity

Whatever criticisms may be made of panic disorder as a diagnosis there is no doubting the clarity and reliability of its main feature, the panic attack. Although the words used in its definition vary there are three features that accompany all panic attacks and are easy to recognise: a sudden onset of symptoms taking place characteristically in the absence of any provoking stimulus (the 'spontaneous' panic attack), the feeling of impending doom or catastrophe, and an accompanying orchestra of unpleasant bodily symptoms (Lader and Mathews, 1970) that may sometimes become the prime feature of the attack. A severe panic attack is remembered with the intensity and clarity of a lover's first kiss, or more prosaically in the words of science, as 'a salient life discontinuity' (Klein and Klein, 1989a). With this degree of accurate recall it is not surprising that the reliability of panic as a symptom is high, with the most conservative measure of agreement (weighted kappa) being as high as 0.9 (Katon *et al.*, 1987; Fyer, 1989).

Given the accuracy of report of panic attacks it might be expected that the diagnosis of panic disorder would show equally good

Table 3.2  Classification of Generalized Anxiety Disorder in DSM-III, DSM-III-R and ICD-10

| DSM-III | DSM-III-R | ICD-10 |
|---|---|---|
| Generalized persistent anxiety of at least one month's duration without the specific symptoms of phobia, Panic or Obsessive–Compulsive Disorder. If anxiety is judged to be due to another mental disorder the diagnosis is not made. Patients must be at least 18 years of age | Diagnosis not made if symptoms 'occur exclusively during the course of a mood or psychotic disorder', but if focus of anxiety unrelated to another Axis 1 disorder the diagnosis can be considered. No age bar | Generalized and persistent anxiety not restricted to any particular environmental circumstances (i.e. is free-floating). Transient (few days only) appearance of other symptoms does not rule out generalized anxiety disorder but diagnosis not permitted if patient has a depressive episode, phobic disorder, panic disorder or obsessive–compulsive disorder |
| Symptoms present from three of the following four categories:<br><br>(i) Motor tension — shakiness, jitteriness, jumpiness, trembling, tension, muscle aches, fatiguability, inability to relax, eyelid twitch, furrowed brow, strained face, fidgeting, restlessness, easy startle | Unrealistic anxiety or worry about two or more life circumstances associated with at least six of the following 18 symptoms:<br><br>A.  motor tension –<br>(1)  trembling (twitching)<br>(2)  muscle tension (aches)<br>(3)  restlessness<br>(4)  fatiguability | Primary symptoms on most days for 'at least several weeks on end'. Symptoms should usually involve elements of:<br><br>A.  autonomic hyperactivity – lightheadedness, sweating, tachycardia, epigastric discomfort, dizziness, dry mouth |

(ii) autonomic hyperactivity – sweating, heart pounding, cold clammy hands, dry mouth, dizziness, lightheadedness, tingling in hands and feet, upset stomach, hot or cold spells, frequent urination, diarrhoea, discomfort in pit of stomach, lump in throat, flushing, pallor, high resting pulse and respiration rate

(iii) apprehensive expectation – anxiety, worry, fear, rumination and anticipation of misfortune

(iv) vigilance and scanning – hyperattentiveness resulting in distractibility, difficulty in concentrating, insomnia, feeling 'on edge', irritability, impatience

B. autonomic hyperactivity –
(5) shortness of breath (smothering sensations)
(6) palpitations or accelerated heart beat
(7) sweating or cold clammy hands
(8) dry mouth
(9) dizziness or lightheadedness
(10) nausea, diarrhoea or other abdominal distress
(11) flushes or chills
(12) frequent urination
(13) lump in throat or trouble in swallowing

C. vigilance and scanning –
(14) keyed up and on edge
(15) exaggerated startle response
(16) difficulty in concentrating or 'mind going blank'
(17) trouble falling or staying asleep
(18) irritability

B. motor tension – restlessness, fidgeting, tension headaches, trembling, inability to relax

C. apprehension – worries about future misfortunes, feeling on edge, difficulty in concentrating

reliability. To some extent this is shown for the diagnosis of agoraphobia with panic, in which kappa values of 0.8 or higher have been reported (DiNardo *et al.*, 1983; Barlow, 1987), but these same authors found that the reliability for the diagnosis of panic disorder itself was lower, at a kappa value of 0.69. On closer examination it appears that the lower reliability for panic disorder relates to the circumstances in which the panic attacks arise, not to failure of their identification. The relative significance of 'spontaneous' and 'situational' panic attacks is discussed with reference to agoraphobia in the following chapter.

There is no other symptom in psychiatry with which panic can be confused. Perhaps the greatest difficulty arises in acute reactions to stress in which the distinction between 'extreme anxiety' and 'blind panic' seem to be more a matter of semantics than any clear distinction in symptoms. However, this difficulty is seldom encountered in practice; the degree of threat is commensurate with the degree of symptoms whereas in the true panic attack they are clearly discordant (Anderson *et al.*, 1984).

The main problems in classification arise from the common link between panic and other symptoms, particularly phobias, and the simultaneous presence of many other symptoms, particularly generalised anxiety and depression. There are difficulties, however, in distinguishing spontaneous from situational panics, which Klein in particular regards as essential in making the diagnosis. This may seem an easy decision to make – a spontaneous attack occurs in the absence of any identifiable stimulus and a situational one is triggered usually by a potentially phobic stimulus – but in practice it is more difficult. Using an event-sampling approach in which patients with panic attacks kept diaries of their attacks and also had their heart rate recorded, the distinction between spontaneous and situational panics was found to be very blurred. Situational attacks were in general more severe, but there was a tendency towards retrospective exaggeration of all episodes. Patients also recorded many attacks as spontaneous even when they occurred in obvious phobic situations (Margraf *et al.*, 1987). These findings cast doubt on the accuracy of patients' accounts of their symptoms and support Marks' (1987b) criticisms of the validity of panic as a diagnostic criterion.

Generalized anxiety disorder is a less clear diagnosis than panic disorder and this is illustrated by the poor reliability of the diagnosis (DiNardo *et al.*, 1983) although this is increased when a structured interview is used (Riskind *et al.*, 1987). Because the criteria for diagnosis consist essentially of long-standing psychological and physical symptoms of anxiety there can also be problems in differentiating generalized anxiety disorder from personality disorder. In particular, the category of avoidant personality disorder in DSM-III-R (anxious in ICD-10) is characterised by persistent tension and social discomfort. Although care has been taken to avoid mood criteria in defining the disorder (avoidant behaviour, restricted lifestyle, hypersensitivity to rejection) there are many similarities between the clinician's concept of chronic anxiety and this type of personality disturbance (Ferguson and Tyrer, 1988) and these are exemplified by the case of Miss Rimms described earlier (case history 3.2).

One of the strongest arguments for separating generalized anxiety disorder and panic disorder is the genetic one. Torgersen (1983) found that concordance rates for anxiety with panic were five times greater for monozygotic (MZ) twins than dizygotic (DZ) twins whereas the concordance rates for generalised anxiety disorder showed no significant MZ-DZ difference. Other data from family studies also support the hereditary aspects of panic disorder (Crowe *et al.*, 1983; Leckman *et al.*, 1983b, Noyes *et al.*, 1986b) and a recent linkage study suggests the identity of a gene locus for panic (Crowe *et al.*, 1987). However, there are some contradictory studies that throw doubt on the specific genetic components to panic and these are discussed in the last chapter of this book.

## Overlap

Panic frequently coexists with other psychiatric symptoms. This has been established for all the neurotic categories in DSM-III (Boyd *et al.*, 1984) but is particularly common in panic disorder. For example, as part of an ambitious project comparing different types of psychological treatment for panic Barlow (1985, 1987) found that of 17 patients with a diagnosis of panic disorder only two (12%) had no other additional diagnosis, a lower proportion than for any of the other anxiety disorders. The most common additional diagnoses were social phobia, simple phobia and dysthymic disorder. Similar proportions have been found by other workers although they have not always used the formal criteria for the diagnosis of panic disorder as before 1980 these did not exist. In the Nottingham study of neurotic disorder (Tyrer *et al.*, 1988b) patients with panic disorder had more additional diagnoses than did those with dysthymic and generalized anxiety disorder (Tyrer *et al.*, to be published). Sheehan's (1983) 'endogenous anxiety' has panic at its core and in his important study in which the effects of antidepressants and placebo were compared as treatments 98% of his population suffered from panic attacks (Sheehan *et al.*, 1980). Symptom co-occurrence was also common and significant degrees of depression, tension, hypo-chondriasis and obsessions were also found in over half of his patients.

It is only by elevating the status of panic in the diagnostic hierarchy that patients can develop the diagnosis of panic disorder. Panic is a gregarious diagnosis: it likes mixing with others and seems to act as a link between other conditions. This does not invalidate its status as a diagnosis, for if panic disorder was like the leader of a pack of wolves and brought in its wake a train of secondary dependent phenomena the diagnosis would be justified. If on the other hand, to extend the metaphor, it is more like one of the flock of sheep which follow each other indiscriminately the justification for the diagnosis disappears.

Although American investigators are quite sure that panic disor-der is a lead wolf a recent meeting of psychiatrists in the United Kingdom led to a consensus statement that adopted a different view. The meeting led to several comments that illustrate scepticism about the primacy of panic, including: 'the natural history of panic either as a cluster of symptoms occurring alone or forming part of another psychiatric illness has not been established'; 'it is unclear whether panic attacks which occur in association with significant generalized anxiety are best considered as a separate disorder or as a more severe form of generalized anxiety disorder'; and although 'panic attacks are often represented as a severe form of more generalized anxiety, it was premature to attempt to describe the relationships between the various symptom clusters' (Ashcroft *et al.*, 1987).

Generalized anxiety disorder also overlaps with other neurotic diagnosis but because in DSM-III it was relegated to the bottom of the hierarchy of classification the diagnosis was only made when other disorders were absent. This gives a spurious impression of separateness, which goes rapidly when the hierarchy is removed as in DSM-III-R.

## Outcome

Both the short- and long-term outcomes of anxiety disorders are controversial issues that are relevant to classification and deserve to be discussed at some length. Whilst it is appreciated that there are several possible outcomes most argument is over their relative frequency. Generalized anxiety disorder and panic disorder have at least five fates, which can be summarised as: (1) resolution; (2) agoraphobia; (3) depressive illness; (4) hypochondriasis; (5) al-

ohol and drug dependence. There are still other possibilities that
so deserve mention.

## esolution

Many patients with panic disorder never progress beyond this
stage. Epidemiological studies in the United States have estimated
the six-month prevalence of panic disorder to be between 0.6% and
.0% (Myers *et al.*, 1984), and only a small proportion of those
ffected need psychiatric contact. Why some, perhaps a clear major-
y, of cases of panic disorder resolve completely is not known. Klein
nd his colleagues (Klein *et al.*, 1980; Klein, 1981) have acknow-
·dged that as most of these patients never see a psychiatrist or even
physician of any sort it is difficult to know what the qualities are
hat lead to resolution. Any knowledge would be most valuable as it
night help greatly in management.

The case history (3.1) given earlier gives some clues. The patient's
rst two panic attacks were 20 years before the second episode and
ad resolved without any professional intervention. It is reasonable
to conclude that the stress created by her husband's infidelity was a
recipitating factor triggering the woman's first panic attacks and
hat the resolution of these attacks was a direct consequence of the
ecision to leave her husband.

Anxiety is always associated with uncertainty and when uncer-
ainty departs anxiety often follows. It is important to remember
hat, in lay terminology, 'panic' describes extremely severe anxiety,
ften amounting to terror, experienced in the face of a major disaster
uch as an earthquake, an aeroplane accident or a raging fire.

The DSM-III adjectives of 'spontaneous situationally pre-
isposed' and 'situationally bound' apply to the diagnoses of panic
isorder and agoraphobia with panic but 'understandable' panic in
uch dramatic situations is almost certainly indistinguishable symp-
omatically. To a lesser degree, attacks of panic occurring only at
mes of severe stress in an individual's life might be expected to
arry a good prognosis and, indeed, they are listed in both major
assifications amongst the stress and adjustment disorders. It is
kely that other influences, particularly constitutional factors and
ast experiences such as separation anxiety, also have an effect on
he resolution of panic disorder. These might affect the cognitive
nterpretation of panic, which may be a key element in both the
ersistence and development of panic into conditions attracting
ifferent diagnoses (Barlow, 1988).

## Agoraphobia

Almost all other outcomes of panic disorder involve secondary elaboration of symptoms, described more evocatively by Stewart Agras (1985a) in his recent book as 'the descent of panic'. Agoraphobia has been postulated by Klein (1981) to be the most frequent diagnostic development and the mechanism of this is illustrated in Figure 3.1.

According to Klein, the 'spontaneous' panic attack, if repeated persistently, 'may also progress, with variable speed, to a set of avoidances. These have the common theme of avoiding situations where if a panic occurs it will be difficult to get help or retreat to home. This set of avoidances, referred to by the misnomer agoraphobia, do not have the common theme of avoidance of public places' (Klein and Klein, 1989b). Persistent avoidance reinforces the development of phobias but does not necessarily resolve the symptoms of panic. During the development of the syndrome of agoraphobia with panic, the panic attacks move through a series of types postulated by Klein from spontaneous to situationally predisposed panics. He uses the notion of 'cueing' to point out these differences: patients at first have no clues as to the cause of their panic but subsequently associate them with some situations more than others.

The accuracy and validity of these subdivisions is open to question as they are based on retrospective data. As noted earlier the work of Margraf *et al.* (1987) throws doubt on patients' accounts of their symptoms; studies that purport to analyse the longitudinal course of panic disorder by retrospective analysis (e.g. Aronson and Logue, 1987) could therefore be seriously flawed.

## Depressive Illness

Significant depressive symptoms can complicate the course of panic disorder. Klein (1981) suggests that demoralisation often precedes these forms of depressive symptoms and is related to the inability to break out of the cycle of panic attacks. However, the degree of depression can be severe and of an 'endogenous' symptom pattern (Uhde *et al.*, 1985). Evidence that depressive episodes may in some way lead to the panic attack comes from the same follow-up study: approximately one-quarter of patients with panic attacks had a major depressive episode either before or within 12 months of the initial panic attack whereas the milder depressions were completely unrelated to panic attacks, and the episodes were often several years apart (Uhde *et al.*, 1985).

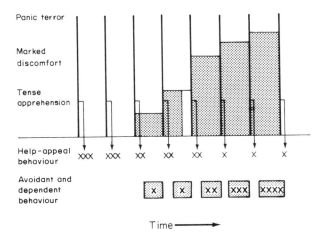

Figure 3.1   Klein's (1981) hypothesis of the development of agoraphobia from panic. (Reproduced by permission of Dr Klein and Raven Press, New York)

In the study of Breier *et al.* (1986) depressive episodes were much less persistent than anxiety symptoms, with 85% of patients with depressive episodes having them temporarily with full resolution in between. Nevertheless, 70% of patients had a major depressive episode during the course of their illness and 43% had their first episode before the onset of their first panic attack.

## Hypochondriasis

Bodily symptoms of anxiety are prominent in panic attacks and if they are the first manifestations of the disorder it is reasonable for patients to assume that they have a physical illness. It is very common for patients to consult their doctors or make their way immediately to hospital casualty departments; the fear of imminent death is one of the important symptoms of a panic attack and emergency action is thought necessary.

Examinations and investigations prove negative but if the panic attacks continue the patient can easily become convinced that something is seriously wrong which the doctors have failed to diagnose. This can then lead to a cycle of referrals to specialist physicians, whose investigations are negative; but the mere fact that they are carried out only reinforces the notion of organic disease to the patient. Perhaps it is surprising that hypochondiasis is not more common in panic disorder; this may reflect the greater sophis tication of patients nowadays, particularly in the United State: where panic disorder has largely been studied. There are good reasons to expect patients who suffer from spontaneous panics to somatise their symptoms because the source of the emotion is unrecognised:

> In normal emotion the subject recognises the provoking stimulus, usually an external one, which gives rise to emotion. He experiences the somatic feelings of physiological arousal, but as he has always detected the source of arousal in regards to the secondary phenomena. In morbid emotion the subject may not recognise the provoking stimulus. He is particularly prone to ignorance if this is an internal psychic one. If he fails to recognise it, the bodily feelings that he experiences are not understood. He is therefore likely to look upon these as primary phenomena and deny the psychic aspects of his condition. Further exposure to the stimulus tends to reinforce initial interpretation of the feelings experienced. (Tyrer, 1973)

The perils of hypochondriasis as a complication of panic are well illustrated by Sheehan (1983) in his book, the *Anxiety Disease*, in which each of the 'seven stages' of panic are given attention in separate chapters. By describing the cause of panic from the stand point of the patient the transitions from one diagnosis to another are seen to be quite rational. Doctors sometimes get irritated with hypochondriacal patients because they do not 'respond to reas surance'. This is not strictly true: reassurance does help but only until the next episode.

> Two days later, she had another bad panic attack that struck out of nowhere. She could not breathe properly and began gasping for air. She was smothering. She knew she was definitely going to die this time. In a flash she lost faith in her doctor. How could he say there was nothing seriously wrong? Here she was dying. (Sheehan, 1983)

It might be expected that panic disorder would also progress readily into somatization disorder, particularly conversion disorder. This complication seems to be relatively uncommon although it has been reported as a complication of agoraphobia with panic (King *et al.*, 1986) and may account for part of the high use of psychiatric services for panic (Boyd, 1986).

The boundaries between hypochondriasis and somatoform disor ders are, as shall be seen in Chapter 6, difficult to draw but perhaps a key element that is lacking in patients with panic disorder is the self dramatic flamboyant advertising of symptoms that is common in the omatoform group. Another concern about hypochondriasis in panic disorder is that it may have some factual basis. There has long been debate over the relationships between anxiety, panic disorder and mitral valve prolapse, a cardiac abnormality that has doubtful pathological significance. Nevertheless, the data from several studies give a rate of 40% for mitral valve prolapse in panic disorder compared with 9% in controls (Agras, 1985b).

Although concern over this association now seems to have been unwarranted, we are still left with one uncomfortable statistic. Coryell et al., (1982) found that patients with panic disorder and agoraphobia with panic (diagnosed retrospectively) had significantly higher mortality from cardiovascular causes of death than the general population, a finding that has remained unexplained. These investigators also found a somewhat higher incidence of suicide in the patients with panic, thus reinforcing the association with depression.

Evidence that the hypochondriasis following panic attacks is directly related to the attacks comes from a study by Noyes et al. (1986a) which showed that successful treatment of panic is associated with reduction of hypochondriacal symptoms.

## Alcohol and Drug Dependence

Alcohol abuse is a recognised problem associated with panic disorder (Sheehan, 1983; Agras, 1985a), but its prevalence is unknown. It has also been established that patients with panic disorder take psychotropic drugs, particularly benzodiazepines, more frequently than do other patients with other anxiety diagnoses (Weissman et al., 1978; Uhlenhuth et al., 1983), and this can also progress to dependence.

Quitkin et al. (1972) have suggested that many patients with alcohol dependence have a history of panic disorder because if this is unresolved and untreated it progresses to both phobic anxiety and alcohol abuse. Successful treatment of the underlying panic and phobias also improves the alcohol problem.

The concept of the person who drinks alcohol to overcome symptoms such as anxiety, the alpha-alcoholic of Jellinek (1960), is now given much less prominence. Nevertheless, there is good evidence that amongst those who drink alcohol to excess there is a considerable minority of anxious, fearful personalities who might well be exposed to panic attacks (Goldstein and Linden, 1969; Løberg, 1981).

## Other Outcomes of Panic

At least two other outcomes figure prominently in panic disorder The first is social phobia as opposed to agoraphobia. If panic attacks are situationally predisposed to occur in social situations it is quite possible for panics to progress to social phobias. Eight per cent of patients with panic disorder were found to develop social phobia in the retrospective study by Breier *et al.* (1986). Preferential avoidance of social situations can therefore lead to a social phobia withou agoraphobia ever rearing its many heads.

Panic can also develop to generalized anxiety. One of the promi nent features highlighted by Klein is anticipatory anxiety in patients who are afraid of having another panic attack. Even if panic attacks never recur, the fear of having one often lasts for a long time anc until the fear goes the patient is tense, apprehensive and may have some of the physical symptoms of anxiety. It is therefore possible for panic disorder to progress to generalised anxiety disorder as a morbid consequence of the panic attacks.

Although each of these consequences is possible and has been documented in various ways the relative frequencies of the different outcomes are unknown. To date there have been no satisfactory *prospective* studies of panic disorder, which is hardly surprising as it is such a recent diagnosis. We must be careful not to infer from retrospective longitudinal studies that the same findings are likely to follow from prospective enquiries, particularly in view of the probable inaccuracy of subjective data. In the Nottingham study of neurotic disorder (Tyrer *et al.*, 1988b) prospective follow-up of 74 patients with panic disorder over a two-year period has so far revealed examples of all the outcomes described above, some tran- sient, some stable, but with no obvious pattern to date. This thus gives support to the notion that panic is indeed 'a common station along the track to other neurotic destinations' (Tyrer, 1986b).

Generalized anxiety disorder has been much less extensively studied than panic. However, it has the same outcomes as panic as it so often precedes panic disorder. For example, in a retrospective study by Cloninger *et al.* (1981) every patient diagnosed as having panic disorder had symptoms of generalized anxiety disorder before their first panic attack; the findings of other studies have been similar (Uhde *et al.*, 1985; Breier *et al.*, 1986). It has also been found that most patients (73%) with generalized anxiety disorder have a history of at least one panic attack at some time in the past (Barlow, 1988).

It is likely that depression is another common outcome of gener-

lized anxiety disorder although this is difficult to determine as in
most of the published work (e.g. Kendell, 1976; Clancy et al., 1978)
panic was not demarcated as a separate disorder and so it is hard to
know how many patients had panic rather than generalized anxiety.

Many patients with generalised anxiety disorder never develop
any further symptoms and remain in a roughly similar state. In such
cases it is tempting to regard the anxiety disorder as a personality
disturbance (see p. 29).

## Treatment

The demonstration that tricyclic antidepressants in the form of
imipramine were beneficial in patients with panic disorder (Klein
and Fink, 1962; Klein, 1964, 1967) was, as described at the beginning
of this chapter, the biggest single stimulus behind the separation of
panic disorder as a diagnostic entity. It represents the first example
of what Klein terms 'pharmacological dissection': the identification
of discrete disorders through their response to drug treatment.
However, close examination of Klein's papers and his writings
establishes that it was agoraphobia with panic that was being
treated with the drug and not panic disorder itself. Thus, Klein
writes:

> The patient with a panic disorder that has not progressed to phobic
> restrictions can be treated succesfully with imipramine. Unfor-
> tunately, there is no controlled study of this specific group since such
> patients usually do not get to psychiatrists but are treated by general
> practitioners and cardiologists. Personal experience with several such
> patients convinced us that their panic attacks respond to antidepres-
> sant medication in exactly the same fashion as those of patients with
> panic disorder that has progressed to a mixed phobia or agoraphobia.
> (Klein et al., 1980, pp. 561–2)

The reason why Klein argued strongly that tricyclic antidepressants such as imipramine were specific for the treatment of panic
disorder and acted by 'blocking' panic attacks was his finding that
these drugs did not reduce secondary anticipatory anxiety or phobic
avoidance. Again, however, it is difficult to be certain of the quality
of his evidence since presumably this was based on personal experience alone or unpublished open studies.

The dangers of relying on anecdotal reports are illustrated by
treatment given to the patient described in case report 3.1. The
patient presented to my psychiatric clinic in primary care with pure
panic attacks without phobic elaboration and had been treated by a
general practitioner five days before I saw her with a low dose of the

antipsychotic drug haloperidol, 1–2 mg daily. Although this type o treatment is not recommended for patients with panic attacks sh had shown marked benefit and so it was continued for two furthe weeks before being withdrawn without any return of panic attacks

It is generally agreed that antipsychotic drugs in low dosage ar ineffective in the treatment of panic and a single anecdote will no contradict this significantly. However, as most of the evidence fo efficacy of drug treatment in pure panic disorder is only at the leve of anecdote even a single case history will carry weight. Severa authors have suggested, again from personal experience alone, tha some patients with panic disorder are 'exquisitely sensitive' to th drug effects of antidepressants, both wanted and unwanted (Klei et al., 1980; Agras, 1985), so that doses as low as 25 mg daily may b effective. If this is so then it suggests that a different pharmacologi cal action from that normally found with antidepressants is involve as it is usual for a higher dose to be given and a considerable perio of time (up to four weeks) to elapse before response is achieved. A alternative explanation is a placebo effect.

By comparison, there is now new data about the success o psychological treatments for panic disorder. Gelder (1986) has re viewed the range of approaches to the study and treatment of pani attacks, and concludes that 'cognitions are abnormal in people wh experience panic attacks and that these cognitions amplify th anxiety response.' Biofeedback is also effective, particularly in ten sion states (Rice and Blanchard, 1982).

Methodologically sound clinical trials have established that vol untary or induced hyperventilation carried out to create a pani attack, but accompanied by cognitive restructuring in which it i explained how panic attacks can be created by misinterpretation o bodily feelings, can provide significant benefit (Clark et al., 1985 Salkovskis et al., 1985; Griez and van der Hout, 1986). Althougl these studies are preliminary they are primarily concerned witl treatment of panic independent of any phobic development. Thi has been extended further by Barlow and his colleagues (Barlow 1988; Barlow and Cerny, 1988), who regard the essential part o treatment as repeated exposure to the somatic symptoms of panic

> At the heart of our treatment program is systematic structured exposure to feared internal sensations. At the outset, patterns of fear are assessed by having patients engage in a variety of exercises designed to produce different physiological symptoms. To activate cardiovascular symptoms, we use exercise. For respiratory symptoms we use voluntary hyperventilation. For audiovestibular symptoms, we induce dizziness. Tension in the chest, which so often signifies an impending heart attack for a panic patient, is produced by tightening

of the intercostal muscles. When feared patterns or combinations of patterns are identified, these become targets for treatment. (Barlow, 1988, p. 451)

Although this technique of 'internal exposure' is interesting it is by no means new and the suggestion that this is a fundamental advance in the treatment of panic is overstated (Waddell *et al.*, 1984). As Barlow acknowledges, the approach has been tried before, most notably by Bonn *et al.* (1971) in an open study in which most of the symptoms described above were induced by lactate injections, a chemical model of anxiety that has achieved staggering popularity since being introduced by Pitts and McClure (1967). Although this technique was of some value in overcoming panic and anxiety it was limited in its effects and was abandoned as a therapy after further unpublished studies (Bonn, personal communication).

There are in any case many similarities between the catastrophising aspects of cognitive therapy in anxiety (Beck *et al.*, 1985) and Barlow's technique of internal exposure (Clark, 1986). Substantial data on the combined approaches being tested by Barlow and his team are not yet available; of particular interest is his study population, all of whom have panic without significant agoraphobic symptoms. The treatment of generalized anxiety disorder is surprisingly similar to that of panic disorder despite the implied distinction in the original formulation of panic disorder as a separate syndrome (Raskin *et al.*, 1982). Thus antidepressants are as effective in generalized anxiety disorder as in panic (Johnstone *et al.*, 1980; Kahn *et al.*, 1986; Tyrer *et al.*, 1988b), and benzodiazepines (with alprazolam in particular) have also been shown to be antipanic drugs (Noyes *et al.*, 1984; Pecknold *et al.*, 1988).

One reason why benzodiazepines were not felt to be effective in the treatment of panic in the early papers may just be related to dosage. It seems likely that all benzodiazepines if given in the equivalent dosage recommended for alprazolam (e.g. the equivalent of 40–70 mg diazepam daily) would be effective in treating panic as well as generalized anxiety (Sheehan, 1987). This goes against Klein's argument for treatment-specific anxiety disorders and supports the view that panic is just a quantitatively more severe form of anxiety than generalized anxiety disorder. Whether it is prudent to give benzodiazepines for panic disorder is another matter. Since the first clear evidence of dependence with therapeutic doses of benzodiazepines (Covi *et al.*, 1974) there is increasing evidence that even short-term treatment for as little as four to six weeks can lead to significant dependence (Fontaine *et al.*, 1984; Murphy *et al.*, 1984b). The treatment of panic with benzodiazepines is not likely to be completed within this timescale and the risks of dependence could well be regarded as unacceptably high.

Despite the many similarities, there may be some distinctions in therapeutic response that need to be addressed. First, beta-adrenergic blocking drugs have been used for the treatment of anxiety, particularly when somatic symptoms are prominent (Granville-Grossman and Turner, 1966; Tyrer, 1976; Tyrer, 1988 for review), but are not effective in the treatment of panic (Shehi and Patterson, 1984). Secondly, the new non-benzodiazepine anti-anxiety drug, buspirone, has anti-anxiety effects in generalized anxiety disorder (Feighner *et al.*, 1982; Rickels *et al.*, 1982) but does not appear to be effective in panic disorder (Rickels, personal communication). Thirdly, relaxation training, while effective when anxiety is generalized, may be less useful in treating panic because the sudden surges of anxiety are too rapid to be brought under control. This is debatable: as with cognitive restructuring and behavioural treatment panic is said by Barlow *et al.* (1984) to be very responsive to treatment.

One common feature about these treatments is the general perception that they are not as powerful in terms of efficacy as other drug and psychological treatments. Again if panic disorder was regarded as a quantitatively more severe form of generalized anxiety (Hoehn-Saric, 1981; Hoehn-Saric and McLeod, 1985) this apparent difference in response could be explained.

## SUMMARY

The separation of panic disorder from other forms of anxiety is an interesting diagnostic hypothesis that has been of great heuristic value. It is now rare to pick up a psychiatric journal (particularly one in North America) without seeing at least one article referring to panic disorder whereas ten years ago the subject was rarely discussed at all. However, the diagnosis is tottering on its pedestal because it has been based largely on studies that have considered it in isolation and do not show it to be fundamentally different from generalized anxiety disorder with the exception of the genetic studies. Moreover, much of the published work concerning pure panic disorder is derivative and anecdotal; the assumption is often made that panic disorder must behave in the same way as agoraphobia with panic, and the largely retrospective work that has been undertaken with this condition is in danger of making it a self-fulfilling prophecy. This may or may not be the case, but without studies on *pure* panic disorder it is difficult to develop satisfactory aetiological hypotheses about the *development* of panic disorder into other conditions if all the evidence comes from one diagnostic population, agoraphobia with panic, which represents only one of the many outcomes of panic disorder.

At the level of simple description panic and generalized anxiety can be distinguished, but their similar response to treatment and longitudinal course suggest that they have many more similarities than differences. Panic is an important symptom but not an exceptional one, and its classification has jumbled the anxiety disorders in a way that has stimulated research but only created puzzlement in the average clinician.

# CHAPTER 4

# Phobic and Obsessional Disorders

Although the cardinal feature of phobias, situational anxiety associated with avoidance, has been recognised for over a hundred years (Westphal, 1871) classification of phobias has altered frequently during this time. Initially psychiatrists seemed more interested in making up names for each phobia depending on which stimulus precipitated fear and avoidance than in studying the cause of the disorder and the handicap produced by it. Thus a host of Greco-Latin epithets ranging alphabetically from acrophobia (fear of heights) to zebraphobia (fear of zebras) was created almost overnight. The classification has always been a compromise between 'lumpers' on one hand, who argue for as few categories as possible, and 'splitters' on the other, who identify large numbers of categories. In the late 1800s the splitters had a field day when new and exciting syndromes were identified in medicine and psychiatry every month. In the case of phobias, however, the splitting has long been shown to make little classificatory sense. Most of the phobias described in this manner belong to one of three groups: the simple (formerly called specific or monosymptomatic) phobias, agoraphobia (literally 'fear of the market place') or social phobias (fear of social situations). Whilst many other conditions have been described as phobias, particularly fears of illness such as cancer or venereal disease (and, more recently, AIDS), these are considered separately in DSM-III-R because they lack the essential element of situational anxiety, although they are mentioned briefly in the section on phobias in ICD-10. In this book they are discussed later in

Table 4.1    Main diagnostic features of phobias in DSM-III-R and ICD-10

| Type of Phobia | DSM-III-R | ICD-10 |
| --- | --- | --- |
| Agoraphobia (with or without history of Panic Disorder) | Fear of being in places from which escape is difficult (when these follow a panic attack or include fear of having a panic attack the diagnosis of Agoraphobia with Panic Disorder is made) | Fear of leaving home, remaining at home alone, entering shops, crowds and public places, or travelling alone in trains, buses or planes (basically similar to DSM-III-R) |
| Social phobia | Fear of being in social situations because of close scrutiny by others and fear of possible humiliation or embarrassment | Fear of scrutiny by other people in comparatively small groups (i.e. not crowds). (Again similar to DSM-III-R, but qualifying statements include the comment 'symptoms may progress to panic attacks') |
| Simple phobia ('specific or isolated phobia in ICD) | Fear of a 'circumscribed stimulus' (object or situation). (Fears of having a panic attack or social humiliation) | Fear of 'highly specific situations' including animals, thunder, flying, darkness, closed spaces, blood etc. Also includes disease phobias (AIDS, venereal disease, cancer) which are not included in DSM-III-R as these are not 'circumscribed stimuli'. (Another difference from DSM-III-R is the comment: 'contact with it (the stimulus) may evoke panic as in agoraphobia or social phobia' |

Avoidance of the defined situation is also described as a common feature in both classifications. Recognition that the fear is unreasonable is also included in the DSM-III-R classification.

connection with hypochondriasis, obsessional and somatoform disorders. The DSM and ICD classifications of phobias are now roughly similar, although the diagnostic category of agoraphobia with panic does not exist in ICD. There are also some important differences in the attribution of diagnoses. As is common throughout the DSM classification, panic is given pride of place. The main differences are shown in Table 4.1. In DSM-III-R any phobic symptoms that develop as a consequence of having a panic attack or of fear of developing panic attacks attract the diagnostic label of agoraphobia with panic disorder, except in the case of social phobia. The other differences between ICD-10 and DSM-III-R are relatively minor: for example, ICD-10 allows panic to occur as a complication of social and simple (specific) phobias and states so specifically.

As there are only small differences between the two major classifications and as the diagnoses of phobic disorder have remained relatively consistent these diagnoses may be thought to be more valid and clear-cut than some of the others discussed in this book. What are the implications of the differences between the three types of phobic disorder in practice? As in other chapters it is useful to examine some case histories to illustrate the three main types of phobia, and to compare them with the related disorder, obsessive–compulsive neurosis.

## Case histories

### 4.1 Agoraphobia

Mr Mulberry was 48 years old and had worked as a clerk in the Civil Service since leaving school at the age of 15. He had always been a methodical and somewhat rigid man and although outwardly friendly had developed few close relationships. He was unmarried and lived alone.

Two years before his psychiatric referral he had been moved to a new post within the Service as a consequence of reorganisation. Although this post was not markedly different from his previous one it was unwelcome and he found it extremely difficult to accommodate to the change. He gradually became more anxious, complained of persistent muscle tension and had difficulty in sleeping. He became gloomy and depressed and saw his general practitioner who prescribed antidepressants in full dosage for several months. Throughout this time he continued to complain mainly of tension and anxiety associated with insomnia. This tension was greatest when he was away from home, either travelling to or from work, and while at work.

Two months before being seen he had an acute panic attack while waiting in the local corner store to pay his weekly shopping. During this attack he had palpitations, shaking of his legs, blurring of vision and dizziness. He was convinced he was going to collapse so he put down his shopping and ran out of the store. He realised that this was a psychological event and did not feel it necessary to consult his general practitioner. He also presumed that the right way of tackling the problem was to go back in the shop again as soon as possible. Unfortunately when he returned again the next day he had a panic attack just at the point of going into the store and again had to return home. A friend was then consulted and offered to get the shopping for Mr Mulberry. Although Mr Mulberry continued to attempt to go into the store on several occasions over the next two weeks he had a panic attack every time and was not able to get beyond the step leading into the store. At about this time he also started feeling panicky when travelling by bus and, as this was not essential to his daily living, stopped using this form of transport. Later this extended further so that he was unable to go to the centre of the city where he lived or mix with large crowds.

When seen at interview he was extremely tense and anxious and described a range of bodily feelings of anxiety in minute detail. At subsequent interviews he was more relaxed and after he had attended on four occasions had little or no anxiety during this time, although his fears of travelling remained the same. It was felt that he would be best helped by a combined approach of relaxation training and gradual exposure to his feared situations. This was carried out with the help of a community psychiatric nurse. Both patient and therapist showed determination in the face of adversity and after a year of treatment he had overcome his avoidance completely. Nevertheless, he remained extremely anxious in his phobic situations and felt exhausted after he had carried out what he continued to regard as 'his tasks'. He was unable to return to work and was made redundant. Two years after treatment his condition was essentially unchanged; his situational fears continued but he had few panic attacks and no avoidant behaviour.

## 4.2   Social Phobia

Mrs Beach was a married woman of 28 with two children around the age of 10. She was referred to the clinic because of her excessive concern over blushing which had led to her avoiding large groups of people. She had left several jobs because she had wrongly thought that her colleagues no longer respected her because she blushed repeatedly in their company. In each of these jobs she had tried to remain anonymous for as long as possible or had become known to only one or two people. Whenever she was better known or greeted in a group she was so convinced she had made a fool of herself by blushing that she could no longer face her colleagues again. She then handed in her notice and waited to get another job until her confidence had improved.

This pattern of behaviour had continued ever since adolescence. As a child she had always felt inferior to her sister and this was reinforced to some extent by her parents who rarely praised and often belittled her. The only time she could ever overcome her sense of inferiority was when she had had a few alcoholic drinks. At these times she was often overconfident and assertive but when she recalled her behaviour the next day she again thought she had made a fool of herself.

At interview she presented as a pleasant and attractive but shy woman. She blushed when describing some of her behaviour and at these times was thrown into confusion. Despite her low self-esteem, there was no evidence of any significant symptoms of depression although she felt gloomy about the future because of the long-standing nature of her problem.

Over the next five years she received a variety of treatments, including antidepressants, anxiety management training, group therapy at a day hospital, attendance at Alcoholics Anonymous (when she became dependent on alcohol for a short period) and anxiety management training together with cognitive therapy. The psychological treatments were the most helpful together with the assertive training she received at the day hospital. By the time of her discharge from care she was symptom-free and had worked in the same job (as a waitress in a high-class hotel) for three years.

## 4.3   Simple (Specific) Phobia

Mrs Nickolan was a 46-year-old happily married woman with no previous psychiatric problems who was referred by her general practitioner because of her fear of snakes. She had always been frightened of snakes but for the first 40 years of her life had lived in Ireland. Ireland contains no snakes, reputedly because St Patrick banished them from the island during the seventh century AD. Since she had come to live in England, however, she had lived in constant fear of encountering a snake and was convinced she would either collapse or have a panic attack if she happened to encounter one. She had never seen a snake although on two occasions when she had seen one on television she was forced to go out of the room.

At interview she presented as a calm, sensitive historian who was reluctant to regard her fear of snakes as abnormal, although she agreed that her preoccupation about encountering one was unnecessary as, without any special avoiding action, she had still not seen a snake in her six years in England.

She was treated by the technique of gradual exposure to the phobic stimulus (i.e. snakes). She could not tolerate the thought of seeing snakes in any form at first and was therefore shown video films of grass snakes and slow worms (both of which are quite harmless) until she felt able to view them with equanimity. Eventually she was confident enough to be taken to see a pet snake (a python) at a nearby laboratory and later made a visit to a zoo where she studied other snakes closely.

After this treatment programme she no longer felt preoccupied and nervous about meeting a snake. When asked to explain why she had improved she maintained that she was still frightened of snakes but that close study of the species that she was likely to encounter in England had convinced her that she could move faster than any of the native species and so could always take avoiding action.

Although she was considered to be cured it is likely that some residue of her phobia persisted because four years later she refused to move to the county of Essex where her husband had been offered a better job because she had heard that adders (the only poisonous snake in England) were occasionally found there.

## 4.4 Obsessive–Compulsive Neurosis

Mr Flewitt was a 38-year-old bachelor who was referred for a psychiatric opinion by his general practitioner because of 'obsessional inefficiency' at work. He worked as a meter reader for the Electricity Board and had reduced his work output by over a half in the previous two years. At interview Mr Flewitt explained that he had to check each meter reading five times and this had led to his reduced output. He had developed this habit gradually over the previous two years but now he could not change it in any way. He was always correct in his meter readings and realised that his multiple checking was unnecessary, but was quite unable to resist the need to continue it. Whenever he checked a reading for a different number of times than five he became anxious and tense and if he forgot the number of times he had made the check he had to start again until he was certain he had done it exactly five times.

He had also become less efficient at home over what he described as his 'silly habits'. These included counting items of cutlery to make sure that none were lost and repeatedly rearranging the contents of drawers so that they were all in neat array. Unfortunately when he closed a drawer he could not be certain that its contents remained undisturbed by the final push required to shut it tight. Often he had to open it again to check the contents, only for his doubts to be repeated when the drawer was closed once more.

He realised his activities were silly and was able to laugh at himself for carrying them out. Indeed, he smiled several times when recounting the stupidity of these actions. He also felt that he alone was responsible for the actions and in no way was he forced to do these by any other influence. On close questioning he admitted that he had always been very pernickety about keeping his possessions and life in order, and also had a tendency to check things more than necessary, but never before in a counting sequence.

He had developed these new symptoms six months after the death of his father. Although he felt he had adjusted to the death emotionally there had been dispute over his father's will and the conflict in his relationship with his two brothers had troubled him a great deal.

At interview he showed no evidence of depressed mood and also seemed reasonably relaxed, although he described symptoms of anxiety when discussing his problems at work. A simple behavioural approach based on response prevention was initiated in which he kept a diary of his anxiety levels and his 'meter reading rate' (numbers of meters recorded per day). He made steady progress, although for a time he could not avoid checking except by writing the meter readings on his hands – only for his anxiety levels to rise again when he ran out of blank skin on which to record the numbers! After six months he had lost almost all his symptoms and was back to his former level of efficiency at work, although still checking more often than he accepted was necessary at home. At discharge an unequivocal diagnosis of obsessive–compulsive neurosis was made.

## AGORAPHOBIA WITH AND WITHOUT PANIC ATTACKS

Agoraphobia, although defined specifically in Westphal's (1871) original paper, covers a diffuse range of situations in current classification. In DSM-III and DSM-III-R agoraphobia is defined in almost identical words and involves: (1) the fear of being in places or situations from which escape might be difficult or in which help might not be available in the event of a panic attack and (2) as a result of this fear the avoidance of such situations or, if confronted, the need for the help of a companion. Typical agoraphobic situations include being outside the home alone, being amongst a crowd or standing in a line, standing on a bridge or travelling by bus, train or car. In agoraphobia with panic disorder the severity of agoraphobic avoidances and panic attacks is assessed. This ranges from mild avoidance (some avoidance but little impairment of lifestyle) through to severe avoidance (nearly or completely housebound). The severity of panic attacks similarly ranges from mild (attacks with less than four symptoms or no more than one panic attack in the past month) to severe (at least eight panic attacks in the past month).

Agoraphobia alone without a history of panic disorder is, as might be expected, identical in all respects to other forms of agoraphobia except that panic attacks are absent. In clinical studies the category is found to be much less common than agoraphobia with panic (Barlow *et al.*, 1986; Barlow, 1988; Klein and Klein, 1989b) and some doubt whether it deserves a separate category. Yet in epidemiological studies agoraphobia without panic is at least as common as agoraphobia with panic (Weissman *et al.*, 1986), a finding that is so much at variance with clinical data that one cannot help thinking that the differences are methodological rather than real (Leckman *et al.*, 1984). The case of Mr Mulberry (case history 4.1), in which the agoraphobia followed a severe panic attack while in his local shop, is typical in its onset and progression and has been described graphically by Klein (1981) and is summarised in the previous chapter (Figure 3.1). Panic progresses to fear of further attacks in vulnerable situations, followed by appeals for support, later leading to agoraphobic avoidance and phobic symptoms.

## SOCIAL PHOBIA

The essential characteristic of this disorder according to DSM-III-R is 'a persistent fear of one or more situations (the social phobic situation) in which the person is exposed to possible scrutiny by others and fears that he/she may do something or act in a way that will be humiliating or embarrassing'. There is quite a range of fears within these situations, including well-circumscribed ones such as fear of vomiting in front of others through to more general fears such as being reluctant to enter social situations in case the person says or does something foolish, exemplified by the case of Mrs Beach (case history 4.2) described earlier.

It is difficult to know why social phobia with panic should not be a perfectly valid diagnosis if agoraphobia with panic deserves such treatment. The DSM-III-R criteria acknowledged this in all but name by commenting that, for example, 'the person with a social phobia of public speaking, and forced to give a talk, almost invariably has an immediate anxiety response, to just feeling panicky, sweating, and having tachycardia and difficulty in breathing'. It is therefore acknowledged that panic attacks and simple phobias may often coexist with social phobia. The implicit assumption in only allowing panic disorder to coexist with agoraphobia as a separate diagnosis in its own right is that the natural course of panic disorder includes the development of agoraphobia. If other phobias develop after the onset of panic disorder this is an associated finding rather than a causal link.

## SIMPLE (SPECIFIC) PHOBIA

Simple phobias, despite the changes in terminology from nominal prefixes to the word 'phobia', through monosymptomatic and specific labels, to the acceptance of the term 'simple', are among the most stable and widely accepted diagnoses in the classification of neurosis. They are well circumscribed, overlap little with other diagnoses and in particular are rarely associated with generalised anxiety (Lader, 1967), and respond extremely well to behaviour therapy involving *in-vivo* exposure to the phobic stimulus (Watson *et al.*, 1971). They also differ from agoraphobia in not responding to antidepressant drugs (Zitrin *et al.*, 1983).

These phobias commonly begin in early adult life and often persist for many years without coming to medical attention. It is only when an event brings the phobia into greater prominence that it causes major concern. Phobic avoidance causes many fewer handicaps in simple phobias than in other phobias because the feared situation is so well defined and usually encountered rarely. The only diagnostic difficulties occur when the phobia is of a more common stimulus. For example, I have had occasion to treat a woman with wind phobia who spent most of her life in a basement flat and refused to come out of doors unless there was absolutely still air. As this meteorological event only took place on about ten days in each year she became as housebound as a severe agoraphobic. If she had experienced panic attacks also she would almost certainly be classified in DSM-III as having agoraphobia with panic attacks.

The recognition that the fear is unreasonable is also part of the DSM classification but not stated specifically in ICD-10. It could be argued that patients with specific phobias only present for treatment if they regard their fears as unreasonable. This issue is discussed in more detail below.

## OBSESSIVE–COMPULSIVE NEUROSIS

This condition (Table 4.2) is the neurotic disorder which has the longest period of consistency in its diagnosis (Janet, 1903). The adjective 'compulsive' now applies to both psychological (ideas, thoughts and images) and motor (impulses and actions) aspects of the condition as these satisfy the diagnostic indications equally. The diagnosis is immediately seen to be superior to many others discussed elsewhere in this book because all the criteria need to be satisfied before the category is formally allowed. The clinician is thus spared the arbitrary lottery whereby a particular diagnosis is decided, for example, by one criterion of a list of seven, when at least four are necessary to make the diagnosis.

There are sometimes difficulties in separating primary obsessional symptoms from those that are secondary to depressive episodes, and there is an understandable tendency for clinicians to identify more depression than may be justified from the clinical presentation as at least depression can be treated more or less satisfactorily. It is often a wise decision also, since many patients are markedly obsessional when depressed and improve dramatically when their depressive symptoms are relieved (Gittleson, 1966).

The alleged compulsions of sexual deviations, drug abuse and activities such as gambling and fire setting are not a diagnostic problem: they are not so intrusive and discomfiting and rarely have the persistence of true obsessions. Similarly, the 'obsessive' desire of the patient with anorexia nervosa to lose weight, the bulimic to binge or the morbidly jealous to spy on the spouse is not a true obsession as it is not resisted as senseless. Indeed, such behaviour is often defended strongly as a necessary and essential activity.

Table 4.2   Diagnostic features of Obsessive–Compulsive Disorder in DSM-III-R and ICD-10

| DSM-III-R | ICD-10 |
| --- | --- |
| Condition characterised by 'recurrent obsessions or compulsions sufficiently severe to cause marked distress, be time-consuming, or significantly interfere with the person's normal routine, occupational functioning, or usual social activities or relationships with others' | Condition characterised by 'recurrent obsessional thoughts or compulsive acts', which are invariably distressing, usually resisted, but which are viewed 'as presenting some objectively unlikely event, often involving harm to or caused by the subject' |
| *Obsessions defined as all of the following:*<br>1. persistent recurrent ideas, thought impulses or images regarded as intrusive and senseless<br>2. attempts are made to suppress or neutralise these obsessions<br>3. recognition that the obsessions are the product of his or her own mind<br>4. the context of the obsession is not related to the symptoms of another Axis 1 (mental state) disorder | *Symptoms present on most days for at least two weeks, and:*<br>1. recognised as own thoughts or impulses<br>2. at least one resisted unsuccessfully<br>3. the thought or act is not pleasurable<br>4. the thought or act must be 'unpleasantly repetitive'<br><br>Diagnosis divided into:<br>(a) predominantly obsessional thoughts and ruminations<br>(b) predominantly compulsive acts (obsessional rituals)<br>(c) mixed thoughts and acts |

## ANALYSIS

### Clarity

Like panic, phobias have an internal consistency that makes them easy to identify. If anxiety is shown only in certain situations, and if these situations can be identified with some accuracy, particularly if they are followed by avoidance, then phobias are present. However, the assumption about all phobias in clinical practice is that they are unreasonable fears and this issue is not addressed satisfactorily in either of the current classifications. For example, it is an unfortunate fact that it is unsafe for women to go out alone in many inner-city streets in some western countries. This is particularly true at night and in many areas is now becoming equally true during daylight hours. Is a woman who lives alone therefore agoraphobic if she refuses to go out of the house between certain hours or is she merely being prudent? The high female to male sex ratio (5 : 1) in agoraphobia may reflect the greater vulnerability of women to assault rather than any intrinsic tendency to develop phobias. Indeed, this point is one of several made by Hallam (1978) in arguing that agoraphobia is merely one form of anxiety neurosis and is only common in women because of their greater vulnerability and more restricted lifestyles in most western societies.

The other problem with agoraphobia is that the situations in which anxiety occurs are not defined clearly. Some people find it hard to accept that agoraphobia can include fear of both open and closed spaces. Similarly, the fear of crowds that is such a handicap in the market place from which the word agoraphobia was derived can co-occur with the fear of being alone (solophobia) within the same disorder. In practice both ICD-10 and DSM-III-R exclude phobias that are only manifested in one situation but this can be an arbitrary decision. For example, a person suffering from claustrophobia may be afraid of travelling by a lift and also in compartments of railway carriages which do not have an outside corridor. The claustrophobia is the same in each instance but because the situations include travelling by public transport and being in an enclosed space the diagnosis of agoraphobia can still be made.

Despite these somewhat semantic difficulties in making the diagnosis, in practice there is good agreement for the diagnosis of agoraphobia with panic but still considerable difficulty in distinguishing it from panic disorder alone. Most investigators can find little difference between patients who satisfy the criteria for both conditions (Thyer *et al.*, 1985, 1987; Noyes *et al.*, 1986b). A past history of separation anxiety is considered by Gittelman and Klein (1984) to be a key feature in predisposing panic patients to the development of subsequent agoraphobia with panic and 18% of patients in a study by Breier *et al.* (1986) had separation anxiety in childhood. However, there was no control group and comparisons between panic disorder and agoraphobia with panic have shown no important differences in the rates for separation anxiety (Thyer *et al.*, 1986). In another study 41 patients with agoraphobia, with and without panic, were compared with 50 normal controls and 83 patients with a variety of neurotic disorders without panic symptoms (mainly eating disorders and obsessive–compulsive neurosis) (Van der Molen *et al.*, 1989). Separation anxiety was found in 17.5% of the agoraphobic group but also in 10% of the normal controls and a high 35.4% of the mixed neurotic sample. Thus the separation–anxiety hypothesis in explaining the aetiology of both panic and agoraphobia receives little support and should be abandoned.

Despite the close similarity between agoraphobia plus panic and panic alone it seems likely that both diagnoses will continue in use. Such is the appeal of panic as a primary diagnosis that it has been suggested that if either diagnosis has to go it should be the agoraphobic one (Noyes *et al.*, 1986b).

Social phobias are also clear-cut and there is usually little difficulty in making the diagnosis. However, in severe cases the person may avoid all situations in which strange people may be encountered. If so, the patient will become as housebound as the agoraphobic and indistinguishable diagnostically. ICD-10 recognises this problem and concludes that in such cases 'if a distinction is very difficult, precedence should be given to agoraphobia' as the diagnosis. One problem that may sometimes give rise to diagnostic confusion is fear of vomiting in public. Although this is reasonably called a social phobia when it is only restricted to social situations, in mild cases it is sometimes difficult to distinguish from a simple phobia.

Simple (specific) phobias are also easy to identify and can rarely cause diagnostic confusion. However, no clear guidelines are given in either classification as to when a condition is a phobia or an understandable fear. For example, there are several studies that suggest that snake phobia such as that described in case history 4.3 is statistically normal as it is found in approximately half the population. Is it therefore right to regard this as a psychiatric diagnosis and would it not be better regarded as part of normal variation? In most instances it is the extent of the avoidance that probably decides whether the condition is pathological and in the case described this was carried to an extraordinary degree and could therefore be regarded as pathological.

The extent of the handicap produced by the phobia is thus often important in deciding whether it is clinically significant. Epidemiological studies have established that the prevalence of simple phobias is high (Lader and Marks, 1971) and it is likely that most of these produce little or no handicap. When pushed to the limit most of us, if we are honest with ourselves, can find some phobic symptom somewhere in the recesses of our psychopathology and often this may be accompanied by avoidance. The dividing line between this and a formal diagnosis of phobic disorder needs to be more clearly defined.

Obsessional disorders are well defined and show greater clarity than almost any other in the neurotic group. This is well demonstrated by the case of Mr Flewitt (case history 4.4) described earlier.

No other diagnosis could realistically be contemplated for his problem of persistent, distressing checking behaviour apart from that of 'atypical' depressive illness developing after the death of his father. The absence of depressed mood, and the lack of any kind of relationship, symbolic or otherwise, between his obsessional symptoms and behaviour following bereavement, makes the distinction an easy one.

### Overlap

There is considerable overlap between social phobias, agoraphobia, depressive illness, panic disorder and generalized anxiety (Boyd *et al.*, 1984; Barlow *et al.*, 1987). This was overcome in DSM-III by the use of a hierarchy in which anxiety was placed on the lowest tier and severe depression on an upper one (see p. 134). Now that co-morbidity is allowed for most disorders in the neurotic category the confusion produced by multiple diagnoses is obvious. Nevertheless, phobic and obsessional disorders have the advantage of consistent patterns of characteristic symptoms *and* behaviour that maintain their separation from the other more diffuse conditions.

The greatest overlapping is with personality disorder. Because phobias and obsessions have persistent behavioural features it is perhaps not surprising that they will overlap with personality disorders, conditions also identified by persistent maladaptive behaviour. As might be predicted, avoidant personality disorder shows the greatest overlap with phobic disorders, and anankastic (obsessive–compulsive) personality disorder the greatest overlap with obsessional neurosis. Thus over 70% of patients with agoraphobia satisfy the criteria for avoidant personality disorder (Loranger, personal communication) and an even higher proportion (75–90%) of obsessional–compulsive patients have a similar type of personality disorder or at least obsessional personality traits (Pollitt, 1957; Kringlen, 1965; Tyrer *et al.*, 1983). This could, however, be a spurious association because phobic and obsessional features, particularly when manifest over many years, satisfy personality disorder criteria also.

There is an increasing tendency to regard patterns of behaviour that have persisted over the recent past (e.g. between two and five years) as representative of premorbid personality (Ferguson and Tyrer, 1988). This tends to improve the reliability of diagnosis but may not be a reflection of true premorbid personality.

# Outcome

One of the strongest arguments put forward to validate the phobic and obsessional diagnostic categories is their persistence over a timescale of several years. Although they show significant degrees of improvement, which is, incidentally, similar in both treated and untreated patients over a five-year period (Agras et al., 1972), they do not tend to change into other types of psychiatric disorder (Pollitt, 1957; Kringlen, 1965).

The likeliest explanation for this persistence is the reinforcing nature of phobic and obsessional avoidance and this is a strong argument for classifying these conditions under a single heading (Marks, 1987c). This does not, however, mean that other conditions do not supervene during the course of phobic and obsessional neuroses. Depressive episodes are common during the course of both agoraphobia and obsessional disorders (Grimshaw, 1964; Mathews et al., 1981; Sheehan and Sheehan, 1983; Breier et al., 1984, 1986) and may further complicate their differentiation from affective disorders at other times. Alcohol abuse may present problems in phobic patients who use the drug for symptomatic relief (Quitkin et al., 1972; Mullaney and Trippett, 1979; Smail et al., 1984) and similar difficulties may lead to dependence on tranquillisers, particularly benzodiazepines (Hallstrom, 1988).

Progression to more serious disorders is rare. Obsessional thinking and behaviour used to be considered as a defence against more catastrophic mental illness, notably schizophrenia (Rosenberg, 1968), but there is no evidence for this outcome from follow-up studies (e.g. Pollitt, 1957; Kringlen, 1965; Marks, 1971).

Compared with panic, generalised anxiety disorder and minor depressive disorders (including dysthymia), phobias and obsessions are much more stable over time (Kendell, 1976; Tyrer, 1986a; Tyrer et al., 1987b). This has also been implied (but not always confirmed as reassessment of diagnosis was often omitted) in long-term follow-up studies of both agoraphobia and obsessive–compulsive disorder (Marks, 1971; Marks et al., 1975; Emmelkamp and Kuipers, 1979; Foa et al., 1987) in which symptomatology of both obsessions and phobias tend to 'run true' over periods ranging from two to four years. This relative persistence gives extra weight to these two diagnoses and might be interpreted as support for panic also, but it is clear from the evidence that it is the agoraphobic part of agoraphobia with panic that is the persisting component. Panic itself changes rapidly and often and shows no persistence unless it is linked to agoraphobia (or, indeed, social phobia).

## Treatment

There are conflicting opinions about the best treatment for phobic and obsessive–compulsive disorders. The only unanimity is shown for simple phobias: behaviour therapy in the form of gradual or rapid exposure to the phobic stimulus is the treatment of choice and other treatments are largely ineffective (Watson *et al.*, 1971; Zitrin *et al.*, 1983). There is no preferred method for exposure and when comparison has been made between self-initiated, therapist-initiated, modelling and flooding approaches the results have been similar (Linden, 1981).

Agoraphobia, both with and without panic, can be treated with desensitisation, exposure treatments (including shaping (Crowe *et al.*, 1972)), various forms of psychotherapy, tricyclic and newer antidepressants, monoamine oxidase inhibitors, benzodiazepines and other anti-anxiety drugs such as beta-blockers. Most of the controversy over their relative merits comes down to the oldest argument in therapy: are drugs or psychological treatments most effective?

The advocates of psychological treatment, of whom Isaac Marks is the best known, argue that exposure treatments are superior when one takes into account all aspects of treatment, including follow-up and the period after withdrawal from treatment (Marks and O'Sullivan, 1989). This opinion is to a large extent influenced by the high incidence of relapse after stopping drug treatment, a finding that seems to be independent of duration of treatment and drug type (Solyom *et al.*, 1973; Telch *et al.*, 1983; Marks and O'Sullivan, 1989), although the related problem of pharmacological dependence is more common with benzodiazepines (Tyrer and Murphy, 1987) and monoamine oxidase inhibitors (Tyrer and Steinberg, 1975; Tyrer, 1984).

Although this is to some extent accepted by the advocates of drug treatment there is a bone of contention between the two parties that has important implications for classification. As might be predicted, it concerns the thorny issue of panic. Tricyclic antidepressants (Zitrin *et al.*, 1983), monoamine oxidase inhibitors (Sheehan *et al.*, 1980, 1984; Buigues and Vallejo, 1987) and benzodiazepines in the form of alprazolam (Sheehan *et al.*, 1984; Ballenger *et al.*, 1988) are all postulated to be effective in agoraphobia because of their antipanic effects. Do exposure treatments work similarly and do drug treatments operate primarily through the medium of panic? The answers are critical in supporting the separation of agoraphobia with panic from agoraphobia without panic disorder (a cumbersome combination of syllables that has attracted the acronym of AWOPD to make it manageable).

There are so many similarities in clinical presentation between panic disorder alone and panic disorder with agoraphobia (Thyer et al., 1985; Noyes et al., 1986b) that only a small change in the diagnostic criteria in the forthcoming DSM-IV would be necessary to create one disorder. Noyes et al. (1986b) suggest that the differences are only ones of severity and as in clinical practice it is rare to se agoraphobia alone the terminology of panic and agoraphobia could be joined. If the effective drug treatments in agoraphobia all oper-ated by 'blocking' panic then there would be a strong case for abolishing agoraphobia as a diagnostic term.

The proponents of drug therapy are in no doubt that panic is 'nodal' and that all other features, particularly avoidance, are secondary (Lydiard and Ballenger, 1987). Exposure treatments only 'help patients to cope with chronic anxiety and spontaneous panics but do not dispel these pathological effects' (Klein and Klein, 1989b, p. 180) whereas antidepressants 'by blocking spontaneous panics foster exposure and decrease avoidance and anticipatory anxiety'. Thus 'rational treatment of agoraphobia consists of (a) education, (b) medication to block spontaneous panics, and (c) then, if neces-sary, structured persuasion to engage in exposure, that may occa-sionally require lessening of anticipatory anxiety by benzodiazepines' (Klein and Klein, 1989a, p. 138). The secondary importance of psychological treatment is very clear from his clinical studies (Zitrin et al., 1978).

The balance of evidence certainly favours the drug proponents with regard to the treatment of spontaneous panic attacks. Such attacks, if genuinely spontaneous in Klein's sense, as opposed to situational panics that can still be subsumed under panic disorder in DSM-III-R, undermine all forms of behaviour therapy (Gelder and Marks, 1966; Marks, 1970) unless they are treated specifically, as for example in the newer cognitive approaches such as those of the Albany group (Barlow, 1988). Unfortunately most of the definitive studies showing the value of exposure treatments did not record spontaneous panic and so it is difficult to find out how much it handicaps response. It is also important to note that panic still improves when exposure alone is given and its 'braking' effect on progress is only a partial one.

If, however, spontaneous panic is not essential to agoraphobia and the behavioural features are primary, exposure treatments become much more important. Despite the finding that agoraphobia without panic is rare in clinical populations there are several epidemiological studies that show it to be much more common in the general population where it may constitute a major-ity of all agoraphobia (Marks, 1987a). The success of exposure therapy is also considerably greater than is suggested by Klein's conclusions, particularly over the longer timescale. What is surprising is that the improvement created by drug treatment does not in itself extinguish the maladaptive phobic and obsessional responses that form the disorder. Stopping drugs after many months or years often leads to relapse. In the case of alprazolam (and other benzodiazepines) this could largely be due to pharmacological dependence (Pecknold *et al.*, 1988), but this explanation is less likely with antidepressants when they are withdrawn slowly, although it still remains a distinct possibility (Bialos *et al.*, 1982; Tyrer, 1984b). Success in confronting both phobic and obsessional situations is more enduring when it is carried out without regular drug ingestion, although when drug treatment is given to 'prime' response to exposure therapy it is sometimes synergistic in its effects (Johnston and Gath, 1973; Ullrich *et al.*, 1975). It is also worth noting that when tricyclic drugs and monoamine oxidase inhibitors have been reported as effective in the treatment of obsessional neurosis (Ananth *et al.*, 1981; Jenike, 1981) there have been no suggestions that they are acting by removing or blocking panics. If panic is 'nodal' in agoraphobia and therefore accounts for response to antidepressants, why is it so conspicuously unimportant in obsessive–compulsive disorders in which response to antidepressants is of the same order as in agoraphobia?

Drug treatment also shows some loss of efficacy over time. This has been shown most clearly with clomipramine in the treatment of obsessive–compulsive disorders. After periods ranging from two to six months of regular treatment there is reduced response although it is difficult to be certain that this is due entirely to the drug. Marks (1983) suggested that drug effects were most prominent in patients who were depressed at the time of initial treatment and that it was wrong to describe the drugs as antiphobic or anti-obsessional. The apparent loss of efficacy after many weeks of treatment (seen most clearly in studies with clomipramine in obsessional patients (Marks *et al.*, 1980, 1988) might therefore be related to improvement in mood so that antidepressant effects are no longer needed. Full analysis of the studies in both agoraphobia and obsessive–compulsive disorders shows that drug effects are broad spectrum and cover more than lowered mood (Marks and O'Sullivan, 1989), so this explanation is unlikely to be true.

In summary, antidepressant drugs and psychological treatments, particularly exposure, have demonstrable efficacy in both phobic and obsessional disorders. Antidepressant drugs (and benzodiazepines in high dosage) alleviate anxiety, panic and depressed mood and this leads to secondary benefits in behaviour. The drugs act quickly but do not maintain their benefits once they are stopped

Table 4.3  Comparison of psychological and drug treatments for phobias and obsessional disorders*

| Diagnosis | Preferred Psychological Treatment | Preferred Drug Treatment | Source |
|---|---|---|---|
| Agoraphobia with Panic Disorder | Exposure therapy | Tricyclic antidepressants | Telch *et al.* (1983); Liebowitz *et al.* (1988) |
| Agoraphobia | Exposure therapy | Tricyclic antidepressants | Marks and O'Sullivan (1989) |
| Social phobia | Exposure therapy, social skills training | Tricyclic antidepressants, monoamine oxidase inhibitors | Ost *et al.* (1981); Liebowitz *et al.* (1985b) |
| Simple phobia | Exposure therapy | None | Linden (1981) |
| Obsessive–Compulsive Neurosis | Exposure therapy | Tricyclic antidepressants | Insel and Johar (1987); Marks and O'Sullivan (1989) |

* The sources quoted are mainly reviews of treatment. Other relevant studies are cited in the text.

and may show some loss of efficacy in long-term treatment. Exposure treatments are slower acting, somewhat impaired in efficacy by coexistent mood disorders, but maintain their improvement. There is less tendency to relapse after stopping treatment.

The relative merits of different classes of drugs compared with exposure treatments in obsessional and phobic disorders are summarised in Table 4.3. Most of the studies with tricyclic antidepressants have used imipramine in phobic disorders and clomipramine in obsessional ones. It is difficult to know whether the choice of antidepressant drug has a bearing on clinical response. Clomipramine acts primarily by inhibiting 5-hydroxytryptamine reuptake and there have been suggestions that selective 5-hydroxytryptamine reuptake inhibitors might have special merit in treating obsessional disorders in particular (Insel and Mueller, 1984). This suggestion is at present based on very weak evidence.

Two studies (Thoren *et al.*, 1980; Ananth *et al.*, 1981) showed clomipramine to be marginally more effective than nortriptyline and amitriptyline respectively in the treatment of obsessive–compulsive disorder, but there was no statistical superiority for treatment effects and only 44 patients were treated in the two studies, with 18 receiving clomipramine. No differences have been found between the effects of clomipramine and other antidepressants in other studies (Rapoport *et al.*, 1980; Mavissakalian *et al.*, 1985).

Despite this negative evidence the new selective 5-hydroxytryptamine reuptake inhibitor, fluvoxamine, has been targeted for the treatment of obsessional disorders. It has predictable positive mood effects but less influence on rituals (Perse *et al.*, 1987).

Monoamine oxidase inhibitors are effective in the treatment of both agoraphobia (Lipsedge *et al.*, 1973) and mixed agoraphobias and social phobias (Tyrer *et al.*, 1973). Phenelzine, when compared with tricyclic antidepressants in the form of imipramine, was better for phobic avoidance and social adjustment but in other respects was similar in efficacy (Sheehan *et al.*, 1980). Similar slight superiority of monoamine oxidase inhibitors over tricyclic antidepressants in treating phobias suggests that the spectrum of treatment for the two classes of drugs shows some important differences (Figure 4.1). There have also been recent reports of the efficacy of monoamine oxidase inhibitors in obsessive–compulsive neurosis (Jenike, 1981) and in view of the close parallel between treatment in agoraphobia and obsessional disorders it is likely that formal clinical trials would confirm their efficacy.

The main concern about benzodiazepines in the treatment of phobic and obsessional disorders is the need to use high dosage and long duration of treatment. These are factors predisposing to dependence (Tyrer and Murphy, 1987) and even after short-term treatment of eight weeks about one in three patients treated with alprazolam for agoraphobia with panic developed an abstinence syndrome on withdrawal (Pecknold *et al.*, 1988). Their value is dubious in view of this risk.

Experience with beta-blocking drugs has been disappointing in agoraphobia and panic and non-existent with obsessive–compulsive disorder. Although beta-blocking drugs such as propranolol in relatively low dosage (e.g. 40–80 mg daily) are effective in situations such as public speaking or playing a musical instrument (James *et al.*, 1977; Brantigan *et al.*, 1982; Hartley *et al.*, 1983) these are best perceived as acute stress situations rather than socially phobic ones (Tyrer, 1988). With more typical (chronic) social phobia and agoraphobia these drugs are of no obvious benefit (Hafner and Milton, 1977) and behavioural treatments are preferred

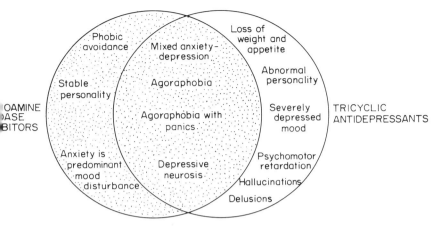

Figure 4.1   Venn diagram showing similarities and differences in the clinical indications for monoamine oxidase inhibitors and tricyclic anti-depressants. (From Tyrer and Shawcross, 1988. Reproduced by permission of the Editors and Publishers of the *Journal of Psychiatric Research*)

(Falloon *et al.*, 1981), although Gorman and Gorman (1987) are enthusiastic about their value in social phobias on the basis of open studies. Only one study has shown beta-blocking drugs to be effective in agoraphobia and then only in conjunction with exposure (Ullrich *et al.*, 1975).

The evidence from treatment efficacy therefore supports the separation of phobias from generalised anxiety disorder. This does not extend to panic disorder as it was noted in the previous chapter that beta-blocking drugs are not usually effective in treating panic.

The results of psychological treatments illustrate the close relationship between obsessive–compulsive and phobic disorders, Marks' (1987c) group of conditions characterised by anxious avoidance. Exposure treatments have almost identical effects in both groups of conditions.

However, other psychological treatments also need to be considered. Barlow has combined behavioural and cognitive elements in his treatment programme for agoraphobia with panic although his main focus of treatment is the panic attack. He favours 'self-based exposure integrated into the personal system of the patient' for the phobic component and 'the psychological approach of exposure to interoceptive cues, accompanied by cognitive therapy and breathing retraining' for the panic component (Barlow, 1988, p. 472). If indeed there were important differences between the outcomes of these two approaches in agoraphobia and panic that supported their specificity, the distinction between agoraphobia and panic as separate disorders would be established. The Albany group are currently studying this and their results will be of great interest.

## SUMMARY

The diagnoses of simple phobia and obsessive–compulsive neurosis or disorder are clearly described and unlikely to be confused with any other neurotic disorder. Their outcome and response to treatment also set them apart from other conditions. Social phobia is also well defined but more information is needed about its outcome and treatment. In particular, it might be expected that behavioural treatments such as assertive therapy and social skills approaches would have specific effects in social phobias alone, but this remains to be demonstrated. Agoraphobia alone is also a clear and unambiguous diagnosis of reasonable clarity although it would be improved if classifiers could decide exactly which situations are truly agoraphobic and which are separate.

Confusion is rife over the diagnosis of agoraphobia with panic, many finding it to be indistinguishable from panic disorder alone, some regarding it as no different from agoraphobia alone and others regarding it as the logical outcome of (unresolved) panic disorder. It is not a good diagnosis, and clinicians should not be allowed to suffer its contradictions for much longer.

CHAPTER 5

# Depressive Disorders

n both ICD-10 and DSM-III classifications depressive disorders are
cluded, together with manic disorder, under the heading of mood
r affective disorders. This completes a major change in the classi-
cation of depressive disorders over the last 50 years. Mood in the
teral sense covers a wide variety of emotions, including anxiety,
nger, ecstasy and irritability as well as depression. Fifty years ago it
as common to regard disorders of mood as all part of one diagnos-
c group:

> There is no need to try and diagnose affective psychosis from psycho-
> genic depression, cyclothymia, anxiety neurosis, neurasthenia, or
> involutional melancholia, these are only sub-divisions of it.
> (Mapother and Lewis, 1941, p. 1860)

ince then we have had the diaspora of mood disorders to all parts
f the globe of classification. Some went to the neurotic disorders
nxiety, depressive and obsessional neurosis), others entered the
ersonality domain (cyclothymia and affective personality disorder)
nd others stayed with the affective psychoses. However, depres-
ion, in one form or another, appears in no less than seven sections
f ICD-9, not only suggesting that it was a common diagnosis but,
ke the chameleon, could present in a multitude of different
olours.

Nevertheless, it was clear that this situation was far from satisfac-
ory and in both major classifications depression has been reined
ack and corralled into one group by nosologists who seem deter-

Table 5.1  Classification of mood disorders in DSM-III-R and ICD-10

| DSM-III-R | ICD-10 |
|---|---|
| Bipolar disorders<br>    bipolar affective disorder<br>    cyclothymia<br>    bipolar disorder (NOS) | Bipolar affective disorders<br>    currently manic<br>    currently depressed<br>    currenly mixed<br>    currently in remission |
| Depressive disorders<br>    major depression, single episode*<br>    major depression, recurrent and<br>        dysthymic disorder<br>    depressive disorder (NOS) | Depressive disorders<br>    severe depressive episode†<br>    recurrent severe depressive<br>        disorder†<br>    mild depressive episode†<br>    recurrent mild depressive<br>        disorder† |
| | Persistent affective disorders<br>    dysthymia<br>    cyclothymia |
| | Other affective episodes<br>    other affective episodes<br>    other recurrent affective<br>        disorders<br>    other persistent affective states<br>    affective disorders (NOS) |

(NOS) not otherwise specified.
* Also includes separate criteria for melancholic and seasonal types.
† Divided into with and without 'somatic' symptoms (see Table 5.2).

mined not to let it escape again. This has been done partly by excluding other disorders of mood although in strict semantic terms the title of 'mood disorders' is incorrect as currently described affective disorders comprise only one part of the spectrum of mood. The appropriate sections in ICD-10 and DSM-III-R should really be titled 'depressive and manic disorders' in order to allow the adjective 'affective' to be applied to other abnormalities of mood also.

There has been a great deal of debate about the classification of depression and much of this has been concerned with the separation of the milder or 'neurotic' depression from the more severe or 'psychotic' ones (Lewis, 1938; Kendall, 1968, 1976). In this chapter most attention will be paid to the milder degrees of depression as these are more relevant to the classification of neurosis.

There is close similarity between the current DSM and ICD classifications of mood disorder (Table 5.1). In the first draft of

CD-10 (WHO, 1987) there was an important difference in that chizo-affective disorders were classified with mood disorders, but n the 1988 draft, as in DSM-III-R, they are coded with the schizo-phrenic disorders.

## SEVERE DEPRESSIVE EPISODE AND MELANCHOLIA

These subjects are not discussed at length in this text because the more severe types of depression are not normally considered to be in the neurotic category. For a disorder to qualify for the description of severe depressive episode or melancholia the patient has to have pathophysiological accompaniments to the depressed mood, including early morning waking, a marked depressive diurnal mood swing and significant appetite reduction with weight loss; in more severe cases psychotic features are present (Table 5.2). In addition this type of depression is usually found in clear-cut episodes with no mental abnormality between illness (and in particular no personality abnormality). It is also associated with a good response to electroconvulsive therapy and other somatic treatments. It is a biological diagnosis through and through: aetiologically, symptomatically and therapeutically. Unfortunately its classification is still open to tremendous controversy: no one doubts that such severe depressive disorder exists but whether it is part of a continuum of depressive disturbance or should be given a 'quality diagnosis' that sets it well apart from other depressive disorders is still not decided. 'Melancholia is one of the great words of psychiatry' wrote Aubrey Lewis in 1934. Great it may have been but at present it is fast losing respect as it shuffles back and forwards across the diagnostic stage, sometimes included but, equally often, excluded as a relic of history.

## OTHER DEPRESSIVE EPISODES

However it is labelled, severe depressive illness is not considered to be among the neurotic disorders, but the milder episodes constitute one of their largest group. Although there are differences in nomenclature between ICD-10 and DSM-III-R, together with a bewildering number of subcategories, their common core is a syndrome of depressed mood, reduced interest, feelings of guilt and worthlessness, agitation (which often appears to be a synonym for anxiety), and concentration and sleep impairment. Two case histories illustrate the more subtle differences between depressive syndromes in this group.

Table 5.2  Classification of Major Depressive Disorder in DSM-III-R and ICD-10*

| | DSM-III-R | ICD-10 |
|---|---|---|
| Main features | *Major depressive episode*<br><br>One or both of the symptoms of depressed mood and loss of interest or pleasure, present for a two-week period | *Depressive episode*<br><br>In typical episodes 'the subject suffers from lowering of mood, reduction of energy and decrease in activity. Capacity for enjoyment, interest, and concentration are impaired, and marked tiredness after minimum effort is common. Sleep is usually disturbed, and appetite diminished. Self-esteem and self-confidence are almost always reduced, and even in the mild form some ideas of guilt and worthlessness are often present; the future seems bleak and suicidal thoughts and acts are common' |
| Operational criteria and diagnostic guidelines | At least five of the following symptoms, including at least one of the first two symptoms:<br>1) depressed mood<br>2) loss of interest or pleasure<br>3) significant weight loss or gain when not dieting (e.g. >5% of body weight in a month)<br>4) persistent insomnia or hypersomnia<br>5) psychomotor agitation or retardation nearly every day<br>6) fatigue or loss of energy nearly every day<br>7) feelings of worthlessness or excessive or inappropriate guilt<br>8) diminished ability to think, concentrate or make decisions<br>9) recurrent thoughts of death, recurrent suicidal ideation without a specific plan, or a suicide attempt or plan to commit suicide | Depressive episodes of any severity may also be accompanied by 'somatic' symptoms, including: '(i) loss of interest or pleasure in activities that are normally pleasant; (ii) lack of reactivity to normally pleasurable surroundings and events; (iii) waking in the morning two hours or more before the usual time; (iv) depression worse in the morning; (v) objective evidence of definite psychomotor retardation or agitation (remarked on or reported by other persons); (vi) marked loss of appetite; (vii) weight loss (often defined as 5% or more of body weight in the last month); and (viii) marked loss of libido. This |
| Severe form | Severe – with psychotic features:<br>i) mood-congruent psychotic features with delusions and hallucinations 'entirely | |

*Severe depressive episode*

Meets the criteria for depressive episode and 'several of the symptoms are marked and distressing, typically the loss of self-esteem and ideas of worthlessness or guilt'. It will 'almost always be found that four or more of the somatic symptoms are present, some of them to a marked degree'. It is unlikely that 'ordinary work, family and social activities' can be continued

Severe depressive episode is further divided into episodes with and without psychotic symptoms, and the latter into mood-congruent and mood-incongruent types which are very similar to the equivalent diagnoses in DSM-III-R

*Depressive episode, moderate severity*

Satisfies the criteria for depressive episode, lasts at least two weeks, 'in which the number and severity of symptoms is such that most subjects will be able to continue normal work, social, and family activities only with considerable difficulty, if at all'

Further subdivided into moderate depressive episode with or without somatic symptoms (four or more symptoms to qualify for somatic group)

(continued on p. 68)

---

nihilism or deserved punishment'

ii) mood-incongruent features include persecutory delusions, thought insertion, thought broadcasting and delusions of control

Severe – without psychotic features: well over five of the above symptoms and marked interference in personal, social and occupational relationships

**Melancholic type**

The presence of at least five of the following symptoms:

1) loss of interest or pleasure in all or virtually all activities
2) lack of reactivity to stimuli which are normally pleasurable
3) depression regularly worse in the morning
4) early morning waking
5) psychomotor retardation or agitation
6) significant anorexia or weight loss
7) no significant personality disturbance before first major depressive episode
8) one or more previous major depressive episodes followed by complete, or nearly complete, recovery
9) previous good response to somatic therapy (e.g. antidepressants, electroconvulsive therapy)

Table 5.2 (contd.)

| DSM-III-R | ICD-10 |
|---|---|
| The depressive episode can also be graded as mild (with few symptoms in excess of those required to make the diagnosis and with little occupational and social impairment) and moderate, in which symptoms are between 'mild' and 'severe' | *Depressive episode, mild severity*<br><br>Satisfies the criteria for depressive episode, lasts at least two weeks, 'but in which the symptoms are neither so numerous nor so severe as in moderate or severe depressive episode. The subject is usually distressed by the symptoms and has some difficulty in carrying on with ordinary work and social activities, but most subjects with an episode of this grade will not cease to function completely'<br><br>Divided into with and without somatic symptoms as for moderate and severe depressive episode<br><br>*Mixed anxiety and depressive disorders*<br><br>A category of mixed anxiety and depression when symptoms are mild and 'neither is clearly predominant'. Can also be coded under 'Other mixed anxiety and depressive disorders' when symptoms or other neurotic diagnoses (obsessive–compulsive, dissociative, multiple somatization disorder) are present but diagnostic criteria for these are not met. Not to be used if the criteria for depressive episode or anxiety disorder satisfied |

# Case histories

## 5.1  Major Depressive Episode

Mrs Measey worked as an office supervisor and had been in the same post for nearly 20 years. In the 18 months before she was referred to a psychiatric clinic the firm had been under threat of takeover and there had been many changes in staff. She felt under more pressure there and was also concerned about her children, aged 18 and 20, leaving home in the near future. One evening when baking cakes she had a sudden feeling of depression and hopelessness and asked herself: 'What am I doing this for? There's no point in trying, I am useless anyway'. She lost all confidence in her ability to work and one week later was unable to go out of the house and was signed off sick from work. She worried all the time, could not sleep at night, continually thought she was doing things wrong, but had no suicidal feelings and no change in her appetite or weight. By the time she saw the psychiatrist two weeks later she was tearful and gloomy but realised that she was depressed and that the feelings at one level of awareness were unjustified. She also recalled a similar episode occurring 15 years earlier without any apparent cause. She was prescribed antidepressants in the form of imipramine 50 mg twice daily. When seen four weeks later she was almost back to her normal self and her self-confidence had returned.

*Diagnosis:* Major depressive episode, not severe.

## 5.2  Dysthymic Disorder

Mrs Whalley, a 56-year-old divorcee, was seen at the clinic after being referred by her general practitioner. He wrote that she 'always seems miserable whenever I see her and I doubt whether much can be done to help her'. At interview she complained bitterly of feeling depressed and maintained that her symptoms began at least 20 years ago although she was unable to remember her age when the symptoms first began. She also noticed that her symptoms were worse whenever members of her family had left home and after her husband died seven years previously she had been extremely depressed with no interest in anything for over a month. Apart from that this time she felt depressed more often than not, often felt tired during the day but could not sleep at night. At interview she showed no evidence of any degree of depression and seemed to enjoy talking about her symptoms at length. Although she had been taking antidepressants from her general practitioner for seven years they had been of no apparent benefit. She was treated with a cognitive approach and her antidepressant withdrawn and although she made significant improvement she remained dependent on the therapist and was reluctant to break off contact entirely.

*Diagnosis:* Dysthymic disorder.

## Cyclothymia

Cyclothymia is also regarded by most clinicians and researc
workers as being outside the spectrum of neurotic disorder. It ha
been a subject of considerable argument by nosologists, as for man
years it was classified among the personality disorders (and still i
under the heading of affective personality disorder in ICD-9). Th
main features are episodic overactivity, expansiveness, and optin
ism that can lead to increased productivity, alternating with gloom
despondency and depression. Close examination has shown tha
this is difficult to equate with personality disturbance. For example
in personal work carried out between 1974 and 1978 to examine th
main types of abnormal personality using cluster analytical tech
niques we were surprised at our inability to find a cyclothymi
group (Tyrer and Alexander, 1979). However, as we were par
ticularly looking at premorbid personality independent of illnes
that was relatively persistent over a long period the absence of
cyclothymic group was perhaps not so unexpected. Cyclothymi
patients regard their mood episodes as abnormal and not part o
their normal personalities and the view now prevails that these ar
more likely to be illness episodes that belong to bipolar affectiv
illness rather than with abnormal personality (Akiskal *et al.*, 1977)
When cyclothymic personality disorder has been identified i
showed poor temporal reliability (Mann *et al.*, 1981b) and this agai
supports the view that it is more a disturbance of mental state tha
one of personality. This view finds expression in both DSM-III-I
and ICD-10.

## Dysthymia

Dysthymia, or dysthymic disorder, was a new addition to DSM-II
and has been further developed in DSM-III-R. It is also bein
introduced in ICD-10. The introduction of dysthymic disorder owe
most to Hagop Akiskal and his colleagues from Tennessee who hav
written extensively about the classification of minor forms of de
pression in studies carried out over the last ten years. Befor
Akiskal's work most minor depressions were classified eithe
loosely under depressive neurosis in ICD or with the personalit
disorders, including affective personality disorder and 'depressiv
personality', a term that has been widely used but which has faile
to achieve formal status is classification (Chodoff, 1972).

According to Akiskal, dysthymia literally means 'ill-humoured
and is characterised by 'an individual who is habitually gloomy
introverted, broody, over-conscientious, incapable of fun and pre

Table 5.3 Classification of Dysthymic Disorder in DSM-III-R and ICD-10

| DSM-III-R | ICD-10 |
|---|---|
| Chronic disturbance of mood involving depressed mood 'for most of the day more days than not', for at least two years. During this two-year period the person is never without depressive symptoms for more than two months | A chronic depression which does not fulfil the description and guidelines of mild recurrent depressive disorder at present (although these may have been fulfilled in the past). Most of the time subjects feel tired and depressed, with lack of enjoyment, finding everything an effort, poor sleep, brooding and complaining, and feeling inadequate, but social function maintained. Such individuals 'are usually able to cope with the basic demands of everyday life' |
| Diagnosis not made if major depressive episode present during the two-year period or if associated with a chronic psychotic disorder | |
| It cannot be established that an organic factor initiated and maintained the disturbance | |
| At least two of the following symptoms present during time of depression: | Diagnostic guidelines include: |
| (a) poor appetite or overeating<br>(b) insomnia or hyperinsomnia<br>(c) low energy or fatigue<br>(d) low self-esteem<br>(e) poor concentration or indecision<br>(f) feelings of hopelessness | (i) longstanding depression of mood, never or rarely severe enough to satisfy diagnosis of recurrent mild depressive disorder<br>(ii) usually beginning in early adult life and lasting for several years, sometimes indefinitely |
| Primary type (no relationship between mood disturbance and non-mood disorder), secondary type (such a relationship is present), and early (before age of 21) and late (on or after age of 21) onset types are all described | |

occupied with personal inadequacy' (Akiskal, 1983). Such patients rarely achieve the diagnostic criteria for major depressive illness (or do so only for very short periods) but tend to be chronically handicapped by their mood disturbance. Because they live and work in the community without having significant contact with psychiatrists except at an outpatient level Akiskal describes them as a major group of 'ambulatory depressions'.

The main features of dysthymic disorder are shown in Table 5.3. The most important criterion for diagnosis is the presence of depressed mood for most of the last two years together with lack of interest over a similar period. At first sight it might appear that such depression must be rare as it is relatively easy to cross the threshold into major depressive disorder, particularly as depressive symptoms only have to be present for two weeks and to be accompanied by a relatively short list of typical symptoms. In our personal research we have found that once patients satisfy the longevity criterion for their depression it is unusual for them not to satisfy the secondary criteria which consist of most of the concomitant symptoms of depression similar to those found in more severe conditions but with rather lower thresholds of detection.

Although in DSM-III-R the synonym for dysthymia is depressive neurosis this is somewhat confusing as dysthymia forms only a small part of the group of conditions that used to be diagnosed as depressive neurosis. Further distinction is made between primary dysthymia, which is not related to a pre-existing chronic disorder, and a secondary type, which follows from a non-depressive disorder such as anorexia nervosa or drug dependence, or a physical disorder such as rheumatoid arthritis. A further distinction is made between cases that develop before the age of 21, described as early onset, and those arising after the age of 21, described as late onset.

The distinction between these types is often difficult, particularly when older patients are seen in whom the onset of the disorder is extremely difficult to identify. The case of Mrs Whalley described earlier (case history 5.2) illustrates this. She was unable to say exactly when her problem began but probably it would be described as late-onset, primary-type dysthymia. Akiskal and his colleagues think that the early-onset primary type is a distinct group that shows important differences from other kinds of dysthymia (Akiskal, 1987).

Dysthymia is particularly difficult to distinguish from major depression because the symptoms are very similar and the criteria of severity used to differentiate them are not obvious ones. The distinction is made more difficult by the frequent coexistence of major depression and dysthymia, commonly called 'double depression'. However, some differences of quality are apparent from Akiskal's own writings. In explaining why chronic mild depression is often missed in clinical practice he points out that many dysthymic patients show little evidence of depression at interview and their symptoms are distorted by their 'demanding narcissistic natures and their almost exhibitionistic flaunting of suffering' (Akiskal, 1983). The doctor therefore assumes that such patients are not genuinely depressed; Akiskal maintains they are. The case of Mrs Whalley (case history 5.2) illustrates this feature, and this may account for the less sympathetic attitude that these patients receive from therapists than those with other depressive disorders.

## Mixed anxiety and depressive disorder

In ICD-10, but not in DSM-III-R, a mixed anxiety–depressive disorder is allowed. It is only a mild disorder and those who qualify for another depressive or anxiety disorder in the classification lose the mixed diagnosis and are given a diagnosis according to the dominant mood in their disorder (and diagnosed as depressive when the clinician cannot make any distinction between the primacy of anxiety and depressive symptoms). Mixed anxiety–depressive disorder is said to be common in primary care and may not come to the attention of doctors at all. Thus it is almost a prologue or a preamble to a diagnosis with implied epidemiological rather than clinical significance.

## ANALYSIS

### Clarity

Although the major symptoms of depressive illness – depressed mood, lack of interest, feelings of tiredness and exhaustion, ideas of guilt and worthlessness – are consistently present in the classification of depression and enable the distinction to be made from other disorders, the subdivisions of depression can hardly be more confused. In DSM-III-R there is reasonable distinction between a severe depressive episode with psychotic features and other types of depressive disorder, but when the psychotic features are not present the distinctions between severe depressive episode, major depressive episode and dysthymic disorder are extremely difficult to discern. They hardly exist at all except in terms of severity, and so the classification as it stands is really a dimensional one in a categorical disguise.

This is a fair reflection of clinical controversy. Although there is now a reasonable acceptance of the existence of a relatively small group of individuals with severe depression associated with qualitatively distinct (psychotic) symptoms (Kendell, 1976) the milder forms of depression have tended to be defined by exclusion. Specific types of depression are identified and all other types, at least until recently in classification, have been placed in the convenient dustbin of depressive neurosis.

It is only in the last ten years that more determined attempts have been made to classify neurotic depression positively instead of only by exclusion. The credit for much of these efforts must go to Akiskal and his colleagues. In one of his early papers on the subject (Akiskal *et al.*, 1978) he pointed out that depressive neurosis not only differed from more severe depression through the absence of psychotic symptoms but was also less likely to be associated with physiological disturbance and more likely to be reactive to circumstances, to be accompanied by other neurotic symptoms such as anxiety and obsessions, and to be associated with personality disturbance. The disturbance of personality was labelled 'characterological depression', a term that has featured frequently in Akiskal's work since and is used to separate two of the major subgroups of neurotic depression (Akiskal *et al.*, 1980). The idea of personality disturbance contributing to the diagnosis of neurotic depression is not a new one and has been prominent in the psychodynamic literature since it was highlighted by Franz Alexander in 1930. Winokur (1987) defines neurotic depression as 'a depression occurring in the context of chronic personality problems or neuroses' and this is confirmed by formal personality assessment of patients with these disorders (which indicates that a substantial minority, close to two-fifths of the total, have abnormal premorbid personalities, mainly of the dependent and obsessional types (Paykel *et al.*, 1976; Tyrer *et al.*, 1983, 1988a). However, although the associated personality disturbance can help to differentiate depressive neurosis from more severe forms of depression, in which, interestingly enough, premorbid personality is more often normal (Tyrer *et al.*, 1988a), it does not help to differentiate the neurotic depressions from other neurotic disorders, in which the prevalence of personality disturbance is similar (Tyrer *et al.*, 1983, 1988a).

In subsequent studies the concept of dysthymic disorder as a low-grade chronic depressive disorder has been generated and is now applied in both the main classifications.

Dysthymia looks to be a way out of the classification impasse at first sight but closer study has shown that it has failed to solve many of the problems. It depends heavily on an accurate description of the depressive disturbance; it is a hard task to recall mood over the previous two years and to decide whether one is depressed 'for most of the day on more days than not' and there is a tendency for reported mood disturbance to be inaccurate. Although the attempt is made in DSM-III-R to exclude more severe depression by avoiding the diagnosis of dysthymia if a major depressive episode has been present during the two-year period this fails to distinguish the condition in practice. Many patients with dysthymic disorder develop episodes of more severe depression (the so-called 'double depression' mentioned earlier) (Frances and Voss, 1987) and it is easy to see from the operational criteria that only a minor change in symptomatology (e.g. continuous symptoms for two weeks instead of for only 12 of the 14 days) can lead to a change in diagnosis. This is not a satisfactory position for any diagnosis.

## Overlap

The major area of overlap for the milder depressive disorders is with the anxiety disorders in their various forms. This is not acknowledged in DSM-III-R in the descriptions of major depressive episode and dysthymia. There is a long list of conditions to be considered under the differential diagnosis of these depressive disorders, including organic mood states, dementias, psychological reactions to physical illness, schizophrenia and schizo-affective disorder. Although it is right to include these conditions because they may present under the guise of depressive disturbance alone it is curious that the anxiety disorders do not merit comment.

Even those who maintain that anxiety and depressive disorders generally can be distinguished without much difficulty acknowledge that the two conditions abut on one another and that differentiating them can be extremely difficult. Using the statistical technique of discriminant functional analysis Roth and his colleagues (Gurney et al., 1972; Roth et al., 1972) were able to distinguish anxiety states and depressive disorders with a very small area of overlap between them. Their results have not been replicated by any other group but have been extremely influential in diagnostic practice. Their contribution is discussed in more detail in Chapter 8 and there is no doubt that their figures demonstrate excellent discrimination. Most other investigators have found a much greater degree of overlap between the two conditions (Mendels et al., 1972; Prusoff and Klerman, 1974; Clancy et al., 1978; Fawcett and Kravitz, 1983; Van Valkenburg et al., 1984; Seivewright and Tyrer, 1989).

Stavrakaki and Vargo (1986) have examined the literature critically and concluded that the differences in findings can be explained to some extent by semantic inconsistencies, methodological and procedural differences, the timing of the disorder in relationship to its course, differences in analysis and the level of interpretation. In general this analysis suggests that overlap is greater in outpatient populations, when the interview is relatively structured and when the interviewer is 'blind' to the original diagnosis. It is also interesting that all investigators find that there is a strong relationship between anxiety and depression but vary in the weight that they give to the importance of this. Thus, for example, using factor analysis Mountjoy and Roth (1982) found that 44% of the variance could be accounted for by a single component measuring severity of illness together with both anxiety and depressive symptoms. A very similar result was found by Mendels *et al.* (1972) but whereas these authors interpreted their finding as evidence of anxiety and depression being part of the same disorder Mountjoy and Roth used the second component of their factor analysis to demonstrate differences between anxiety and depression and thus missed the first component.

Unfortunately much of the argument over the degree of overlap is at a level of debate that is not familiar to the average clinical psychiatrist. In practice, however it is interpreted, anxiety and depression walk hand in hand through all settings where psychiatry is practised and diagnostic systems have to take account of this.

Milder depressions, particularly dysthymic disorder, overlap with personality disorder, as Akiskal has frequently pointed out. In DSM-III-R dysthymic disorder is said to be particularly common in people with borderline, histrionic, narcissistic, avoidant and dependent personality disorders. It is interesting that a depressive mood disorder has not been identified in the second axis of classification in DSM-III. In personal research (Tyrer and Alexander, 1988, pp. 53–5) we have identified a subgroup of personality disorders in which the characteristics of feelings of worthlessness, shyness, aloofness, sensitivity and conscientiousness are most prominent and which is best described as dysthymic personality disorder. It is extremely difficult to differentiate between this and a chronic mood disorder such as dysthymia if the condition has extended over many years, in some cases throughout adult life.

As already mentioned, the difficulties in differentiating between dysthymic disorder and major depressive episode are considerable as both share the same qualitative features and differ only in terms of severity.

## Outcome

In general the outcome of single depressive disorders is good, and it is not surprising that the more chronic disorders subsumed under dysthymia tend to be more persistent (Akiskal *et al.*, 1980; Seivewright and Tyrer, 1988). Sometimes the disorder begins late in adolescence and persists throughout most of adult life, exemplified by the case of Mrs Whalley described earlier (case history 5.2), and in such cases it is difficult to know whether the diagnosis should be that of a mental state or personality disorder. Akiskal (1989) makes a strong case for describing cyclothymic, hyperthymic and depressive temperaments but regards them as precursors of chronic mood disorders rather than alternative conditions.

The outcome of other depressive disorders is more favourable, at least in the short-term. Criticism can be made that the threshold of identification of major depressive episode is too low, so that many conditions not regarded by most clinicians as 'true' depressive illness are included under its label. If so, it could explain the apparent failure of biological markers of depression such as the dexamethasone suppression test to detect such depression and predict response to treatment (Carroll, 1985). In particular, the short duration of symptoms necessary to meet the initial criteria (two weeks) results in the inclusion of many who would not be regarded as significantly depressed in clinical practice. If depressed mood and lack of interest have been present continuously for two weeks it is relatively easy for the condition to accumulate the remaining criteria for the diagnosis. Many people are depressed for two weeks or longer as a natural response to loss and adjust to this without specific intervention, DSM-III-R acknowledges one condition within this group, 'uncomplicated bereavement', but there are many others also.

At the other extreme there is an unfortunate abundance of evidence that chronic depressive disturbance is not only widespread (Cooper, 1965; Shepherd *et al.*, 1966; Myers *et al.*, 1984; Robins *et al.*, 1984) but also ignored and poorly treated (Weissman and Klerman, 1977; Keller *et al.*, 1982). This goes some way towards explaining the need for a chronic depressive category in classifications, although the implied equivalence of dysthymic disorder and the older term, depressive neurosis, is unfortunate. The separation of single from recurrent depressive episodes in ICD-10 is also likely to have been influenced by the poorer outcome of the latter group, although the fact that past course is the only satisfactory way of predicting prognosis is indicative of the poverty of other clinical criteria.

When long-term outcome is considered the findings are bleak. Lee and Murray (1988) found in an 18-year follow-up study that 95% of patients admitted with depression had at least one relapse in this period, which supports the view of Angst *et al.* (1973) that all patients with affective disorder will relapse if followed up for long enough. In Lee and Murray's (1988) study patients had been allocated to a position on the psychotic–neurotic continuum by R.E. Kendell at the time of admission; the outcome showed that the psychotic patients were more likely to be readmitted and to fare worse over the longer timescale. The authors concluded that this 'provides further longitudinal validation of the distinction between neurotic and psychotic depression'.

As depression is a treatable condition doubts have also been expressed about the quality of the differences between the chronic and acute forms of depressive illness. The differences could easily be explained by inadequate treatment of the chronic group only (Keller *et al*, 1982).

The different outcome of anxiety states and depressive illness has been a major influence on classification. Even if there is substantial overlap between the symptoms of anxiety and depression this is of little importance if the two diagnoses can be separated in prognostic terms. The results, unfortunately, show no consistent picture. In an early paper Walker (1959) found that anxiety states (including phobias) had a better prognosis than other affective disorders, particularly when they presented suddenly and with no obvious precipitants.

Two of the 1972 series of papers from Newcastle concentrated on outcome and reported different findings. Anxiety states showed consistently poorer outcome over a four-year period than depressive illnesses (Kerr *et al.*, 1972; Schapira *et al.*, 1972). Details of treatment over this period were not included. Snaith (1981) points out that this was a major omission as treatment could have influenced the outcome quite independently of the original diagnostic differences. At the time these studies were carried out the most common treatments were benzodiazepine tranquillisers and hypnotics for anxiety disorders and antidepressants for depressive disorders. Subsequent studies (see below) have shown that this separation was incorrect and that long-term benzodiazepine treatment is both hazardous and relatively ineffective. If, therefore, treatment had followed diagnostic practice the patients with anxiety states would have improved less than those with depression, but this would be explained by the effects of treatment only.

The way in which the follow-up results were expressed by Schapira *et al.* (1972) is also open to misinterpretation. Percentages of patients showing significant improvement were described rather than absolute levels of pathology. If patients with anxiety states and depressive illnesses constituted a single syndrome, in which anxiety was more prominent at lower levels of severity and depression at higher levels, then the apparently worse outcome of the anxiety group would be expected. The depression group could remain the same or improve over follow-up whereas the anxiety group would also have the potential to get worse. In personal work we found strong support for this view (Tyrer *et al.*, 1987a,b). Patients with a diagnosis of anxiety neurosis had fewer symptoms and better social

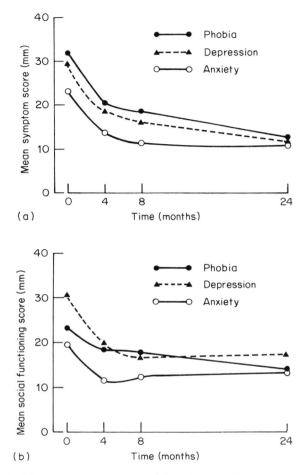

Figure 5.1    Mean symptom scores (a) from Present State Examination and social functioning scores, (b) from the Social Functioning Schedule (Remington and Tyrer, 1979), in patients with phobic anxiety (*n* = 16), depressive neurosis (*n* = 51) and anxiety neurosis (*n* = 11) after 4, 8 and 24 months. (From Tyrer *et al.*, 1987b. Reproduced by permission of the Editor of the *British Journal of Psychiatry*)

functioning than those with depressive or phobic neurosis. They did not improve as much as the other patients during a two-year follow-up period but the levels of pathology of all three diagnoses were similar at the end of this period (Figure 5.1).

In many ways it is to be expected that there is significant overlap between anxiety and depression in all psychiatric classifications. Patients often make different interpretations of mood states than do psychiatrists (Leff, 1978), and, as in the last resort the patients' views carry the most weight, some confusion between anxiety and depression reflects clinical reality and should not need apology. When Jane Austen writes of Mrs Bennett, 'when she was discontented she fancied herself nervous', how would the independent psychiatrist describe her state? I would wager that some would find her to be depressed, and some anxious, and not a few would find evidence of both emotions, and the opinions would be little different even if DSM-III-R and ICD-10 were given in their most structured forms!

When significant degrees of anxiety and depression coexist in what otherwise appears to be a primary depressive disorder then the outcome is much less satisfactory than when depression dominates the clinical presentation (Van Valkenburg *et al.*, 1984; Stavrakaki and Vargo, 1986). This is consistent with epidemiological evidence that major depression with an anxiety disorder is associated with higher rates of similar disorders in first-degree relatives than major depression alone (Leckman *et al.*, 1983a; Noyes *et al.*, 1986). This is an important point in favour of a separate category for mixed depressive and anxiety disorders and is discussed at greater length in the last chapter of this book.

## Treatment

More work has been carried out on the relationship between the treatment and classification of depressive disorders than of any other neurotic disorder. The introduction of antidepressant drugs 30 years ago stimulated a great deal of enquiry into all forms of treatment and was also a powerful stimulus to improved methodology of clinical trials in psychiatry. Before the introduction of antidepressant drugs there were no satisfactory research studies proving the worth of any psychiatric treatment for depression. Since then the general methodology introduced to investigate the therapeutic benefits of antidepressants has been extended to cover the range of treatment, including analytical psychotherapy (Weissman, 1987).

The results have supported the separation of mild depressive illness (neurosis) from severe illness (psychosis, or melancholia) to some degree (Bielski and Friedel, 1976) although not nearly to the extent predicted by those who originally championed the distinctions between endogenous and neurotic depression (Kiloh *et al.*,

1972). For more severe depressive illness (usually requiring inpatient treatment) electroconvulsive therapy is the most effective treatment (Medical Research Council, 1965; Morris and Beck, 1974; Avery and Winokur, 1977), particularly when given in bilateral form (Gregory *et al.*, 1985). Tricyclic antidepressant drugs follow closely in terms of efficacy (Liebowitz, 1985; Lipman *et al.*, 1986), with monoamine oxidase inhibitors faring little or no better than placebo (although the early studies may have used too low a dosage for too short a time) (Ravaris *et al.*, 1976; Tyrer, 1979).

Psychological treatments are not effective in the most severe forms of depressive illness but, mainly in the form of cognitive therapy, are as effective as antidepressants in the milder forms of depression (Rush *et al.*, 1977; Blackburn *et al.*, 1981; Murphy *et al.*, 1984a; Teasdale *et al.*, 1984). Preliminary results from the recently completed large-scale National Institute of Mental Health study in the United States organised by Parloff and Elkin, in which cognitive therapy was compared with interpersonal psychotherapy, placebo and imipramine, show the effects of all active treatments to be very similar (Weismann, 1987; Klerman, 1988). Interpersonal psychotherapy is focused on current depressive problems and thereby shares much with cognitive therapy and much less with analytical approaches. Because it is relatively straightforward it is well suited to treatment in primary care, where it has already proved its worth (Klerman *et al.*, 1987). It, too, has been shown to be of similar efficacy to amitriptyline in depressive episodes and over a timescale of a year led to better social functioning than did drug treatment (Weismann *et al.*, 1976). However, there are no suggestions in any of these studies that there are subgroups of depressive disorders that respond differently to these treatments, which would be necessary if they were to influence classification.

Monoamine oxidase inhibitors are of equivalent efficacy to tricyclic antidepressants in depressive neurosis (Paykel *et al.*, 1982). The difference in the efficacy of monoamine oxidase inhibitors between the mild and severe forms of depression has no satisfactory pharmacological explanation, and is an empirical finding that squares with other evidence that their anti-anxiety effects are somewhat greater than those of tricyclic antidepressants (Kelly *et al.*, 1970, 1971; Lipsedge *et al.*, 1973; Liebowitz *et al.*, 1984, 1985). In the milder forms of depression it is uncommon not to find anxiety as a significant coexisting symptom and this may affect response to monoamine oxidase inhibitors.

There is greater evidence of differences in the efficacy of treatments between mild and severe depressive illness than between neurotic depression and the anxiety disorders. As has been made

Table 5.4  Effects of treatment and diagnosis in the Nottingham study of neurotic disorder

| Rating Instrument | Diagnosis | Mean Percentage Change (0–10 wk) | | | | |
|---|---|---|---|---|---|---|
| | | Diazepam (n) | Dothiepin (n) | Placebo (n) | CBT (n) | SH (n) |
| CPRS (total score) | Dysthymia | 10 (10) | 23 (11) | 9 ( 7) | 23 (23) | 20 (12) |
| | GAD | 6 (10) | 33 (10) | 26 ( 9) | 25 (25) | 21 (11) |
| | Panic | 9 ( 7) | 21 ( 7) | 24 (10) | 20 (32) | 31 (17) |
| | Total (95% CI) | 8 ( 0, 16) | 27 (19, 35) | 21 (13, 29) | 22 (17, 27) | 25 (18, 32) |
| MADRAS (depression score) | Dysthymia | 10 | 27 | –16 | 28 | 21 |
| | GAD | 9 | 35 | 30 | 23 | 21 |
| | Panic | 9 | 26 | 30 | 21 | 34 |
| | Total (95% CI) | 10 ( 0, 20) | 30 (20, 40) | 18 ( 8, 28) | 23 (17, 29) | 27 (19, 35) |
| BAS (anxiety score) | Dysthymia | 5 | –6 | 6 | 17 | 15 |
| | GAD | 13 | 36 | 19 | 22 | 20 |
| | Panic | 12 | 13 | 17 | 21 | 29 |
| | Total (95% CI) | 10 ( 1, 19) | 14 ( 5, 23) | 15 ( 6, 24) | 20 (15, 25) | 22 (14, 30) |

| HADS | | | | | | |
|---|---|---|---|---|---|---|
| (depression self-rating) | Dysthmia | -3 | 11 | 5 | 22 | 15 |
| | GAD | 5 | 26 | 13 | 29 | 9 |
| | Panic | 5 | 14 | 24 | 17 | 25 |
| | Total (95% CI) | 2 (-7, 11) | 17 ( 8, 26) | 15 ( 6, 24) | 22 (17, 27) | 18 (11, 25) |
| HADS | | | | | | |
| (anxiety self-rating) | Dysthymia | 7 | 14 | 2 | 15 | 11 |
| | GAD | 10 | 24 | 19 | 20 | 10 |
| | Panic | 18 | 13 | 12 | 15 | 25 |
| | Total (95% CI) | 11 ( 4, 18) | 18 (11, 25) | 12 ( 5, 19) | 16 (12, 20) | 17 (12, 22) |

CI, confidence interval.

The figures represent the mean percentage change after ten weeks treatment in: total symptomatology – measured by the Comprehensive Psychopathological Rating Scale (CPRS), an observer-rating scale (Åsberg et al., 1978); depression – measured by the Montgomery and Åsberg Rating Scale for Depression (MADRAS) Montgomery and Åsberg, 1979) and by the Hospital Anxiety and Depression Scale (HADS), a self-rating scale (Zigmond and Snaith, 1983); and anxiety – measured by the Brief Scale for Anxiety (BAS) (Tyrer et al., 1984) and by HADS.

There were 201 patients with data suitable for analysis (numbers in parentheses). Those receiving additional treatment were also included; more of those allocated to placebo had these during the ten-week period.

Diazepam was less effective in all groups. Diagnosis had no significant influence on response to treatment (all values $P>0.1$).

(From Tyrer et al., 1988b. Reproduced by permission of the Lancet.)

clear from other chapters in this book, antidepressants and mono-amine oxidase inhibitors are equally effective in panic, generalised anxiety, dysthymia and major depressive episodes. Attempts have been made to formulate a diagnosis of 'atypical depression' specifically responsive to monoamine oxidase inhibitors ever since the first report of their value by West and Dally (1959). Although this has met with some success (Robinson *et al.*, 1978; Liebowitz *et al.*, 1984, 1985) the concept of atypical depression remains diffuse and a recent review of its characteristics (Paykel *et al.*, 1983) concluded that it has little classificatory value.

## Nottingham Study of Neurotic Disorder

No formal comparisons have been made between the effects of drug treatment and cognitive therapy in panic, generalised anxiety and depressive disorders in a single design apart from the Nottingham study of neurotic disorder. This showed no diagnostic differences in outcome between an antidepressant drug (dotheipin), a benzo-diazepine (diazepam), cognitive and behaviour therapy, and a self-help treatment package after ten weeks of treatment (Tyrer *et al.*, 1988b) (Table 5.4). Diazepam was less effective in all diagnostic groups, supporting other evidence that despite the benefits of short-term treatment (Chouinard *et al.*, 1982) these become less over time (Shapiro *et al.*, 1983) and compare unfavourably with antidepressants in both anxiety and depression (Kahn *et al.*, 1986; Lipman *et al.*, 1986). An 'intention to treat' model was used in which all patients entered into the study had their results analysed even if they received additional treatment during this period. Those allocated to placebo treatment received significantly more additional treatment (31%) than the other groups and this contributed to the generally good outcome in this group also.

Studies of this nature are difficult to mount because of the relatively large number of subjects required. It is also difficult to remove the effects of bias when psychological and drug treatments are being compared, when at the most only single-blind procedures can be employed. However, in the Nottingham study the assessors (all trained psychiatrists) were unaware of both initial diagnosis and treatment received when they made their assessments as all patients were asked not to discuss any aspect of treatment with the research doctors.

If these findings are replicated dysthymic disorder should be classified with the anxiety rather than depressive conditions with respect to treatment. Its independent status should be reviewed.

*Psychological Treatments*

The findings of similar efficacy of psychological treatments in the anxiety and depressive disorders is not as surprising as it might appear at first sight. Although it might be thought that there would be important differences in the treatment approaches for these conditions it is interesting to note their many similarities. Thus Teasdale (1985), writing about depression, summarises the mechanism of action of successful treatments in this way: 'effective psychological treatments for depression reduce "depression about depression" by reducing its aversiveness and increasing its perceived controllability'. Barlow (1988, p. 473), in discussing his psychological treatment model for panic, emphasises that 'cognitive and breathing control procedures, and perhaps relaxation procedures as well, instil a sense of control over negative events that are otherwise perceived as uncontrollable'. The two statements could be transposed without any change in meaning, and other focused anti-anxiety treatments such as anxiety management training (Butler *et al.*, 1987) could easily be adapted for depressive disorders.

More disturbingly for cognitive theory, the finding that self-help was as effective as cognitive therapy (at least in the first ten weeks of treatment) in the Nottingham study suggests that either the successful elements of treatment are not dependent on significant cognitive restructuring or, if they are, this can be achieved by a straightforward approach that promotes independence along the lines of the highly successful home-based and self-treatment approaches with phobic patients (Jannoun *et al.*, 1980; Mathews *et al.*, 1981; Marks *et al.*, 1983; Ghosh and Marks, 1987).

## SUMMARY

In summary, response to treatment of depressive illness supports a distinction between a small group of disorders variously termed melancholia, severe depressive episode or delusional depression, and a much larger group with milder symptomatology (including the somewhat misleadingly named major depressive episode (DSM-III-R), single and recurrent mild depressive episodes, and dysthymia. Within this group with mild symptoms there is no support for differential response in dysthymic disorder compared with the other depressive disorders. There are also many examples of similar response to treatment in both mild and moderate depression and the anxiety disorders. Neither pharmacological nor psychological dissection of treatment has been useful in identifying or confirming the division of anxiety and depressive disorders that remains a fundamental part of the classification of neurosis. This is a worrying issue that deserves further attention and is examined later in this book.

CHAPTER 6

# Somatoform and Dissociative Disorders

This group of conditions used to be collectively known as hysteria. Although the concept of hysteria has changed many times from the original notion of the 'wandering womb' creating affliction by malposition in other parts of the body it has always retained the simulation of physical illness as a core feature. What has caused dispute throughout the ages is the mechanism by which the symptoms of hysteria are created. This is the main reason why somatoform and dissociative disorders have been separated in both major psychiatric classifications and why hysteria has been abolished as a diagnosis. In the dissociative group there are clear-cut psychosocial stressors that have a major bearing on the form and outcome of the disorder whereas these features are lacking in somatoform disorders. The conditions can be viewed as being at opposite ends of a spectrum with regard to these features (Figure 6.1).

The definition of hysteria in the twentieth century is best summarised by a memorandum from the Medical Research Council published to aid the assessment of war neuroses:

> Hysteria is a condition in which mental and physical symptoms, not of organic origin, are produced and maintained by motives never fully conscious directed at some real or fancied gain to be derived from such symptoms. (Medical Research Council, 1941)

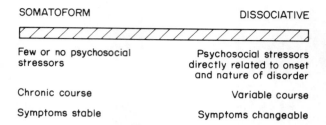

SOMATOFORM                                         DISSOCIATIVE

Few or no psychosocial                    Psychosocial stressors
stressors                                       directly related to onset
                                                  and nature of disorder

Chronic course                                      Variable course

Symptoms stable                                 Symptoms changeable

Figure 6.1   Classification spectrum of 'hysteria' in ICD-10 and DSM-III-R

This pithy statement encapsulates the combination of disease simulation and unconscious gain that is essential to the term. More wordily and prosaically, hysteria was described in ICD-9 in 1978 as:

> Mental disorders in which motives, of which the patient seems unaware, produce either a restriction of the field of consciousness or disturbances of motor or sensory function which may seem to have psychological advantage or symbolic value. It may be characterised by conversion phenomena or dissociative phenomena. In the conversion form the chief or only symptoms consist of psychogenic disturbance of function in some part of the body (e.g. paralysis, tremor, blindness, deafness, seizures). In the dissociative variety, the prominent feature is a narrowing of the field of consciousness which seems to serve an unconscious purpose and is commonly accompanied or followed by a selective amnesia. There may be dramatic but essentially superficial changes of personality sometimes taking the form of a fugue (wandering state). Behaviour may mimic psychosis, or, rather, the patient's idea of psychosis. (World Health Organization, 1978)

Although most of these elements are still present in the revised classifications the notion of 'unconscious purpose' has been avoided because it cannot be measured and fails all the requirements of an atheoretical descriptive system. The reader will note from the following pages that the determination to keep out the unconscious is at times only achieved by linguistic tortuosity.

Although somatoform and dissociative disorders lie on the same spectrum they are worth examining separately. Whilst dissociative disorders are all recognisable as conditions that came under the heading of 'hysteria' in former classifications the somatoform group includes many conditions that would formerly have been diagnosed as depressive, anxiety or personality disorders.

## SOMATOFORM DISORDERS

This group of conditions will appear strange to many readers who are otherwise familiar with the terminology of psychiatric classification. The essential feature of this group is the presence of physical symptoms concerned with somatic function for which no organic cause can be found. The symptoms are persistent but usually involve several organ systems either simultaneously or consecutively and this may often serve as a pointer towards a psychiatric rather than a physical diagnosis.

The reasons for this form of symptom expression are not specified in the revised classification and, in particular, the symbolic and dynamic interpretation of the symptom formation is avoided. As noted in Chapter 2 the word 'neurosis' was eliminated from the American psychiatric classification (except in parenthesis) in 1980 primarily because of its (unfounded) assumption that unconscious motivation played a part in symptom formation. The new diagnoses attempt to confine themselves to descriptive, measurable criteria so that good reliability and better understanding are achieved.

Unfortunately in the case of somatoform (and dissociative) disorders this purity of purpose is difficult to uphold. There are many thousands of potential patients with physical symptoms for which no obvious cause can be identified but who nonetheless have a physical rather than a psychiatric diagnosis. The key features that make the doctor suspect a psychiatric diagnosis are the association of the symptoms with abnormalities of mood, their changing nature and the suspicion that the patient is deriving some benefit from the symptoms. Thus although there may be considerable disability produced by the symptom (primary loss) this is to some extent compensated or more than overcome through the advantages gained.

Involvement of these concepts has to admit, at least implicitly, the notion of unconscious motivation. Indeed, it is the principal component of classification, because if the physical symptoms are controlled by the person concerned (i.e. faked) the condition is diagnosed (in DSM-III-R) as a factitious disorder or malingering. Thus the classification of this group has to fall back on the use of psychological constructs that are currently impossible to measure and verify.

In the past most patients with somatoform disorder would have been described as having conversion hysteria. Hysteria has long been a psychiatric diagnosis, reaching its heyday in the late nineteenth century when the French neurologist, Charcot, used to demonstrate gross examples of conversion symptoms (*la grande hystérie*) to large appreciative audiences at the Saltpêtrière Hospital in Paris. Charcot (1889) regarded hysteria as a neurological condition and its return to psychiatry was achieved by two of his pupils, Breuer and Freud (1893). They showed that many cases of hysterical conversion could be helped through the technique of abreaction, by exposing and releasing the conflicts allegedly giving rise to the hysterical conversion. This observation was the germ from which Freudian psychoanalysis grew and subsequently extended with less justification to encompass the whole of psychiatric disorder.

The diagnostic concept of hysteria has been through many vicissitudes since Breuer and Freud's original paper. Freud broke with Breuer when he suggested that the cause of the hysterical conflict was almost universally a sexual one. He subsequently found in his clinical practice that almost every patient he interviewed had hidden sexual experiences, usually of an incestuous relationship with a parent. Freud was naturally reluctant to admit that the respectable middle-class Viennese were universally incestuous and was rescued by his postulation of the Oedipus complex. By suggesting that boys were sexually attracted to their mothers and girls to their fathers he was able to extricate himself from a difficult theoretical position; the explanation was that those who claimed incestuous relationships under psychoanalysis were not necessarily telling the truth: they were only reflecting the wish to have a sexual relationship with the parent as this was a basic urge.

In the 1920s and 1930s when Freudian theory was at its peak of influence large numbers of neurotic patients were diagnosed as suffering from hysteria, and sexual conflict was usually regarded as its cause. In both World Wars there were many examples of both dissociative and conversion hysteria brought on by the stress of battle in the front line. After scandalous ignorance of this in the First World War, when many sufferers were imprisoned and some shot on the grounds of desertion of duty, the condition was recognised readily and in the Second World War it responded well to abreactive techniques, both with and without drug assistance (Sargant and Shorvon, 1945). Subsequently the diagnosis came under threat again when evidence from peacetime studies suggested that the condition showed poor consistency, had no genetic predisposition and, most damningly, that many patients with an original diagnosis of hysteria subsequently developed a definite organic illness, usually a neurological one (Slater and Glithero, 1965). Thus the diagnosis of hysteria was 'a disguise for ignorance and a fertile source of clinical error. It is in fact not only a delusion but a snare' (Slater, 1965), and should therefore be abandoned.

Although the diagnosis of hysteria continued to be used for the next 15 years it has weakened its hold and may slip off altogether.

Table 6.1   Classification of somatoform disorders in DSM-III-R and ICD-10

| DSM-III-R | ICD-10 |
|---|---|
| Body Dysmorphic Disorder (dysmorphophobia): preoccupation with imagined defective appearance without the belief being of delusional intensity. | Dysmorphophobia not classified among somatoform disorders and not included as a term in this classification |
| Conversion Disorder: the loss of, or alteration in, physical functioning suggesting a physical disorder in which psychosocial stresses 'apparently related to a psychological conflict or need' are temporarily related to the initiation or exacerbation of symptoms | Included under dissociative disorders (p. 104) |
| Hypochondriasis: preoccupation with the fear of having, or the belief that one has, a serious disease without evidence of this on physical evaluation | Hypochondriacal syndrome: persistent preoccupation with a possibility of having one or more serious and progressive physical disorders, manifest by persistent somatic complaints |
| Somatization Disorders: recurrent and multiple somatic complaints of several years duration, for which medical attention has been sought, but which are not due to any physical disorder. The disorder begins before the age of 30 and has a chronic but fluctuating course | Multiple somatization disorder: multiple, recurrent and frequently changing physical symptoms, which usually have been present for several years and which are associated with a long and complicated career through both primary and specialist medical services |
| Somatoform Pain Disorder: preoccupation with pain in the absence of adequate physical findings to account for the pain or its intensity | |
| Undifferentiated Somatoform Disorder: similar to Somatization Disorder but does not reach the 'full symptom picture of Somatization Disorder' | |

Although Slater's work had a major impact the body blow came from an alternative diagnostic approach in the United States (Hyler and Spitzer, 1978).

This was pioneered by Samuel Guze and his colleagues at the

Washington University School of Medicine in St Louis. They found that an apparent form of conversion hysteria, the presentation of many physical symptoms from several organ systems, showed great temporal consistency, had a pattern of development and variation unlike any organic disease, and was almost invariably found in females. Examination of the literature revealed that a French physician had written about a very similar population a hundred years previously (Briquet, 1859) and so Guze's team generously gave the title of Briquet's syndrome to this group of disorders. This has been the main stimulus behind the development of the concept of somatoform disorders. Physical symptoms can be described and reported in some detail and the behaviour of patients presenting with them can also be identified without difficulty. Using this information different subgroups of somatoform disorders can be identified. The introduction of the term has been as American initiative and ICD-10 has been, somewhat reluctantly, carried in its wake. Somatoform disorders are not present in any existing ICD classification but have been incorporated into ICD-10 (Table 6.1).

Before describing the classification of somatoform disorders in more detail it is useful to examine two clinical cases that illustrate the differences between somatoform and dissociative disorders. The examples chosen illustrate the course and development of symptoms as well as the main clinical features. These have a greater influence on diagnosis than in many of the other neuroses, a positive development that could be taken up with profit by those involved in classification generally.

## Case histories

### 6.1  Somatization Disorder

Mrs Mackie was a housewife aged 55 who was first referred to a psychiatrist when she was 32. The initial referral letter from her general practitioner had a note of despairing appeal,

> Please can you do something for this woman. She has been in and out of my surgery for years with one minor complaint after another. Sometimes its her arthritis, sometimes her bowels, and sometimes her palpitations and her heart. I've never been able to find anything physically wrong with her and all tests at the hospital have been negative. It makes no difference what I and the hospital say, she keeps coming back and is never satisfied. She seems miserable all the time but insists she is not depressed. Has she an inadequate personality?

When first seen by the psychiatrist she was said to be depressed and was treated with antidepressants – more in hope than conviction as the doctor concerned agreed with the general practitioner that she was a 'chronic inadequate whittler'. The drugs had little effect apart from helping her to sleep better, but for this reason she continued to take them. Some years later she was prescribed benzodiazepines when she became extremely tense and worried about her continued symptoms and could not sleep. Again the benefit of these drugs was limited but it required great effort on the part of her general practitioner to withdraw them, and then it was achieved only through substitution by low-dosage thioridazine, a sedative antipsychotic drug.

Each time there was a major event in her life (mainly her daughters leaving home) she complained more about her symptoms. At the age of 48 she was found to have myxodoema and treated with thyroxine. This diagnosis was greeted with enthusiasm by both general practitioner and patient as it was felt that now a physical 'cause' had been found her troubles would all be over. Unfortunately it was not to be and after a few months Mrs Mackie's old symptoms returned in full force.

When seen in the clinic ten years later she talked at great length about the pains in her body caused by all 'the bones rubbing against each other', vibratory sensations in all body orifices and gripping sensations in her stomach and bowels. There were no signs of depression at interview although she complained that at times she lost energy and could not see the end of her troubles except through death.

She was treated at first by a psychotherapeutic approach designed to help her to understand the reasons behind her fluctuation in symptoms. This included exploration of her feelings when her daughters left home and her understandable resentment and feelings of rejection. Her medication was also reduced to doses that had virtually no pharmacological action but which she insisted were necessary to keep her well. Although there was some improvement in her symptoms she remained very preoccupied with her bodily complaints and continued to consult her general practitioner every two months.

## 6.2   Complex Dissociative Disorder

Mr Brown was 45 and worked as a part-time clerk in a building firm. He did not earn much, but as his wife had a well-paid job as a personnel officer and their two children had grown up and left home this was not a problem. At times in the past he had stopped working in order to look after the children and take on household responsibilities, so working only part-time was not a problem for him. It also gave him more opportunity to carry out his preferred work as an unpaid deputy treasurer of a social club. He was on the club committee and was well respected for his work.

The club was concerned with a deprived inner-city area that was very short of leisure activities and, by providing the resources for bingo sessions, dances, lunch meetings for pensioners and discos for younger members, the committee was a major integrating force in the community.

Mr Brown enjoyed this work immensely; his clerical experience was a help in keeping the books in order and his responsibilities were well within his capabilities. More importantly, he was a figure of substance in the community whereas at home he sometimes felt inferior to his more capable wife.

This cosy picture was disturbed by Mr Brown's colleague, the club treasurer, who suddenly disappeared from the area taking £3000 of the club's funds with him. The police were informed and interviewed all members of the committee. All of them were cleared of any involvement in the theft. However, Mr Brown continued to worry about it and blamed himself for failing to detect that the treasurer was not to be trusted. He had problems getting to sleep and found it difficult to concentrate.

Three weeks later his behaviour suddenly changed. He appeared to be unaware of his surroundings and talked in an odd staccato voice, repeating statements and phrases unnecessarily and inappropriately: 'I must talk to Mrs Gould' (another committee member), 'It is clear' and 'My wife stays with me' were the most frequent. His general practitioner made a diagnosis of 'psychosis' and asked a psychiatrist to visit. At assessment he appeared like an automaton, staring ahead with glazed eyes and repeating the same three phrases. He refused to let his wife leave the room during the examination and held her arm continuously.

He agreed passively to come to a day hospital immediately, provided that his wife was allowed to come also, although agreement was obtained non-verbally as he would not utter any words apart from his three phrases. He was sedated with diazepam and placed in a quiet room. It was felt that his condition was a dissociative reaction to the problems at the club and an abreactive technique was used to explore his feelings further.

He was taken back over his recent experiences, the psychiatrist recounting them in chronological order and making suggestions about his likely feelings when the facts of the theft became known. He became extremely angry, rose from his couch and smashed his fist into the door, shouting incoherently as he did so. He needed to be restrained by six nursing staff and it was impossible for anyone, including his wife, to communicate with him in any form that suggested understanding. He was admitted to a residential psychiatric hospital the same day.

The next day he was apparently well and completely recovered from his experiences, apart from a painful and swollen right wrist joint. He could not remember any of his experiences from the previous three days. The next day he was discharged and continued to be seen as an outpatient. He remained well but four months later he suddenly became depressed with morbid thoughts about his responsibilities. After a short course of anti-depressant drug treatment and day hospital support he felt much better and, more significantly, was able to recall and express his feelings about the theft at the club without any distress. Six months later he was well and free of symptoms.

These cases are from opposite poles of the somatoform–dissociative spectrum. The first satisfies the criteria for the diagnosis of somatization disorder, a long-standing concern with various bodily complaints of no physical basis, and the second is a complex dissociative disorder involving motor and mental function. The first is chronic, unprecipitated and remarkably persistent in its major symptoms; the second is clearly related to a traumatic event, has a good prognosis and changes in its presentation over time. The late development of depressive symptoms is a consequence of the original stresses but quite different from the initial manifestations.

Although these cases could not by any stretch of the imagination be regarded as part of the same condition there are difficulties with some of the intermediate disorders. It is also fair to say, at least in the United Kingdom, that somatoform disorders have not achieved respectability in clinical settings. Certainly in my experience, when the collective title is introduced in case discussions it is almost done so 'in parentheses' and often with embarrassment.

One of the major problems in allowing somatoform disorders the status of a separate diagnostic group is that there is still some doubt as to whether conditions formerly described as hysterical disorders deserve to be excluded by giving them a diagnosis among the somatoform group. This implies the absence of significant psychosocial stressors (with the exception of conversion disorder in DSM-III-R) even when the clinician feels they are present. There is particular difficulty with those disorders in which conversion symptoms and dissociation are present simultaneously. There are other difficulties in classifying disorders that do not have the same temporal links with psychosocial stresses but that none the less have common physical symptoms (e.g. panic). These difficulties are more freely acknowledged in the ICD-10 classification which appears to include somatoform disorders as a distinct group with some misgivings.

## Body dysmorphic disorder (dysmorphophobia)

In this condition there is either excessive concern over an imagined abnormality of appearance or grossly exaggerated concern over a minor abnormality that would not be noticeable to most people. Most commonly this refers to the size or shape of the nose, to facial blemishes such as wrinkles, freckles or moles, or to deviations in the shape of the mouth, jaw, eyes or of other parts of the body that are at least partly visible, such as the feet, legs, arms or breasts. Although in the past this condition has been labelled 'dysmorphobia' this is inconsistent with the policy of regarding phobias as situational anxiety associated with avoidance; thus in DSM-III-R this terminology has been dropped (but replaced by equally cumbersome polysyllables). The main diagnostic criterion for body dysmorphic disorder is the abnormal preoccupation with the imagined or exaggerated defect but the belief has to be of non-delusional intensity. In addition if the abnormality only occurs in association with anorexia nervosa and transexualism then the diagnosis is not made.

In ICD-10 this condition is not classified separately with the somatoform disorders but, if present, is included under the heading of hypochondriacal syndrome unless the abnormal belief is sufficiently strong to be regarded as a delusion, in which case it is included under the heading of delusional disorder. This difference probably reflects the long-standing view in European psychiatry that patients with dysmorphophobia belong with the schizophrenias rather than the neurotic disorders.

The condition looks out of place with the others included in the somatoform disorders. There is considerable doubt about its relationship with psychosocial stressors but what is clear is that it does not have the clear-cut antecedents of most dissociative disorders. However, as concern about the shape or prominence of the nose is such a common symptom in this disorder it is not surprising that psychodynamically orientated psychiatrists have drawn an obvious symbolic parallel with another organ! The other concern is that although the symptoms in this condition refer to bodily appearance they do not have the same status as the bodily symptoms of other disorders in the somatoform group. It seems likely that the condition will continue to be classified under labels such as monosymptomatic hypochondriasis (Bishop, 1980), schizophreniform disorder, or a delusional syndrome in addition to the classification currently recommended.

## Conversion disorder

This condition is only included in DSM-III-R in the somatoform disorders. Because of its alternative title 'hysterical neurosis, conversion type' it is included in the dissociative disorders described later.

## Hypochondriasis

This condition, with its extended terminology of hypochondriacal neurosis and hypochondriacal syndrome, is similarly described in both classifications. Although it is well recognised as a symptom there has often been concern about its status as a diagnosis (Barsky and Klerman, 1983). Hypochondriasis is a common symptom in schizophrenic and depressive illness and although it shows internal

onsistency of symptoms (Brown, 1936) there have been sugges-
ons that it should be abandoned as a diagnosis because it so often
o-occurs with other symptoms, the most notable being depression,
vhich should take precedence in diagnostic description (Kenyon,
965). Nevertheless, when all forms of secondary hypochondriasis
re stripped away one is still left with a core of 'essential' hypo-
hondriasis which cannot be explained by any other diagnostic
escription (Bianchi, 1973).

The characteristic feature of hypochondriasis is the concern that
ne has, or might have, a serious physical disease because of the
xperienced bodily symptoms. Not surprisingly, doctors are con-
ulted early in this condition and by the time patients reach psy-
hiatric attention they have usually had several consultations with
lifferent doctors together with abundant reassurance that no sig-
ificant disease is present. Although this reassurance is sometimes
ffective in the short term, it seldom persists and most patients
ontinue to be concerned that the physician either has missed a
erious illness by inadequate diagnostic assessment or alternatively
las found out that the patient has a serious illness and will not
lisclose the information. As might be expected, the symptoms that
ften attract attention are anxious ones such as awareness of the
ast-beating heart, dizziness or gastrointestinal symptoms.

The operational criteria in DSM-III-R include: (1) the preoccupa-
ion with serious disease, (2) the absence of any physical diagnosis
n 'appropriate physical evaluation' and exclusion of symptoms
vhich are those of panic attacks, (3) the persistence of concern
about the alleged or feared disease despite medical reassurance,
4) the persistence of the disturbance for at least six months and
5) the belief that one has a serious physical disease (if present) is not
f delusional intensity. Similarly, in ICD-10 two diagnostic
uidelines are given:

> (1) A persistent belief that the patient has one or more serious
> physical illnesses 'even though repeated investigation and examina-
> tions have identified no adequate physical explanation',
> (2) persistent refusal to accept medical advice and reassurance.
> (World Health Organization, 1988)

The main difference between ICD-10 and DSM-III-R is that the fear
f having a serious physical illness is included under hypo-
hondriasis in DSM but not in ICD. Another of the phobias, illness
hobia or nosophobia, is also included under this heading.

The hypochondriacal disorders exemplify one of the underlying
leficiencies of classification in the somatoform group. The diagnosis
s essentially a negative one; the patient has symptoms at a certain

Table 6.2  Classification of Somatization Disorder in DSM-III-R and ICD-10

| DSM-III-R | ICD-10 |
|---|---|
| A. A history of many physical complaints or a belief that one is sickly, beginning before the age of 30 and persisting for several years.<br><br>B. At least 13 symptoms from the list below. To count a symptom as significant, the following criteria must be met:<br><br>(1) no organic pathology or pathophysiologic mechanism (e.g. a physical disorder or the effects of injury, medication, drugs, or alcohol) to account for the symptom or, when there is related organic pathology, the complaint or resulting social or occupational impairment is grossly in excess of what would be expected from the physical findings<br>(2) has not occurred only during a panic attack<br>(3) has caused the person to take medicine (other than over-the-counter pain medication), see a doctor, or alter life-style<br><br>**Symptom list:**<br><br>Gastrointestinal symptoms:<br><br>(1) **vomiting (other than during pregnancy)**<br>(2) abdominal pain (other than when menstruating)<br>(3) nausea (other than motion sickness)<br>(4) bloating (gassy)<br>(5) diarrhoea<br>(6) intolerance of (gets sick from) several different foods | *Multiple somatization disorder*<br><br>The main features are multiple, recurrent and frequently changing physical symptoms, which usually have been present for several years before the patient is referred to a psychiatrist. Most patients have had a long and complicated career through both primary and specialist medical services, during which many negative investigations or fruitless operations may have been carried out.<br><br>*Diagnostic guidelines*<br><br>A definite diagnosis required the presence of all of the following:<br>(i) at least two years of multiple and variable physical symptoms for which no adequate physical |

(i) persistent refusal to accept the advice or reassurance of several different doctors that there is no physical explanation for the symptoms;
(iii) some degree of impairment of social and family functioning attributable to the nature of the symptoms and resulting behaviour.

Symptoms may be referred to any part of the body, but gastrointestinal sensations (pain, belching, regurgitation, vomiting, nausea etc.) and abnormal skin sensations (itchings, burnings, tingling, numbness, blotchiness, soreness etc.) are among the commonest. Sexual and menstrual complaints are also common.

Marked depression and anxiety are frequently present, and may justify specific treatment.

The course of the disorder is chronic and fluctuating, and is often associated with longstanding

(continued on p. 100)

Pain symptoms:

(7) **pain in extremities**
(8) back pain
(9) joint pain
(10) pain during urination
(11) other pain (excluding headaches)

Cardiopulmonary symptoms:

(12) **shortness of breath when not exerting oneself**
(13) palpitations
(14) chest pain
(15) dizziness

Conversion or pseudoneurologic symptoms

(16) **amnesia**
(17) **difficulty swallowing**
(18) loss of voice
(19) deafness
(20) double vision
(21) blurred vision
(22) blindness
(23) fainting or loss of consciousness
(24) seizure or convulsion
(25) trouble walking
(26) paralysis or muscle weakness
(27) urinary retention or difficulty urinating

Table 6.2 (*contd.*)

| DSM-III-R | ICD-10 |
|---|---|
| Sexual symptoms for the major part of the person's life after opportunities for sexual activity:<br><br>(28) **burning sensation in sexual organs or rectum (other than during intercourse)**<br>(29) sexual indifference<br>(30) pain during intercourse<br>(31) impotence<br><br>Female reproductive symptoms judged by the person to occur more frequently or severely than in most women:<br><br>(32) **painful menstruation**<br>(33) irregular menstrual periods<br>(34) excessive menstrual bleeding<br>(35) vomiting throughout pregnancy | disruption of social, interpersonal and family behaviour. The disorder is far more common in women than in men, and usually starts in early adult life.<br><br>Dependence upon or abuse of medication (usually sedatives and analgesics) often results from the frequent courses of medication. |

**Note:** The seven items in boldface may be used to screen for the disorder. The presence of two or more of these items suggests a high likelihood of the disorder.

time but no explanation can be found for them. I once worked for a physician who took all his patients' symptoms seriously at first but if subsequent investigations all turned out to be normal the diagnosis of 'hysterical hypochondriasis' was pinned firmly on the unfortunate patient. This type of label is difficult to shake off and yet it is well established that many such individuals develop an organic disease subsequently (Gatfield and Guze, 1962; Slater, 1965). In retrospect the initial presenting symptoms could have been regarded as a prodrome of the illness rather than independent and psychological in origin.

Another problem is that many patients who show true hypochondriasis are simultaneously suffering from a physical disease although the symptoms complained of by the patient are not those of the disease concerned. Nevertheless, it takes a bold doctor to diagnose which symptoms are false indicators of psychological origin and which are genuinely caused by an organic disease.

An additional problem is that patients suffering from hypochondriasis may be excessively sensitive to changes in their bodily functions and may therefore perceive correctly changes that others would not detect. This has been shown for at least one common symptom, awareness of heart beat (Tyrer *et al.*, 1980), although it does not extend to somatic symptoms such as muscle tension (Tyrer and Lee, unpublished).

## Somatization disorder

As already mentioned, the stimulus behind the separation of somatoform disorders as a separate diagnostic group came from psychiatrists from the Washington University School of Medicine in St Louis under the guidance of Samuel Guze and encouraged by Eli Robins. Somatization disorder is the jewel in the somatoform crown and far more work has been carried out into the clinical features, prevalence, diagnostic stability and outcome of this disorder than for the rest of the somatoform group together. This explains the detailed operational criteria necessary to make the diagnosis; Mrs Mackie's case (case history 6.1) represents a good example. A series of studies from St Louis established in the 1960s that Briquet's syndrome, as it was then called, was a reliable and stable diagnosis when it was identified in women, had an onset before the age of 35 and usually much earlier, and was characterised by bodily symptoms from several different organ systems, but notably the gastrointestinal and reproductive ones (Perley and Guze, 1962; Guze, 1967; Guze *et al.*, 1971b; Woodruff *et al.*, 1971; Cloninger *et al.*, 1984) (Table 6.3).

Table 6.3   Other characteristics of Somatization Disorders

| Feature | DSM-III-R | ICD-10 |
|---------|-----------|--------|
| Onset | Usually begins in the teens | Usually begins in 'early adult life' |
| Course | Chronic and fluctuating, rarely remits for longer than a year | 'A long and complicated career through both primary and specialist medical services' |
| Sex ratio | Somatization Disorder is described as very rare in males whereas Undifferentiated Somatoform Disorder is more common in males but still much less common than in women | 'Far more common in women than men' |

This combination of persistent somatic complaints beginning early in life and being too diffuse to explain by organic pathology has been reproduced in ICD-10 without significant alteration although the 'symptom checklist' required to make the diagnosis is omitted and the diagnosis couched in more general terms.

## Undifferentiated somatoform disorder

The undifferentiated somatoform (and somatization) disorders reflect the fact that many people having persistent somatic complaints with no organic basis do not satisfy the very strict criteria for the diagnosis of full somatisation disorder. This group is larger than the one with the full syndrome and does not show the almost exclusive female predominance in somatisation disorder.

## Somatoform pain disorder

Pain is distinct from any other symptom and is probably a more frequent bodily complaint than almost any other. Somatoform (formerly called psychogenic) pain disorder is similar to undifferentiated somatization disorder except that pain is the only symptom. Unfortunately it can apply to a large number of people, many of whom have, or will subsequently prove to have, an organic cause for their pain. It is a condition that lacks clear identifying criteria and, unlike somatisation disorder, the symptoms are not multisystem and relatively easy to separate from organic disease. The clinical notion of secondary gain is often conspicuously lacking (although of course it is not a criterion for making the diagnosis). Most other symptoms in somatoform disorders can in principle be tolerated but pain is an exception. As Merskey (1979, p. 119) puts it: 'Why choose a symptom which hurts?' Often the condition begins after acute tissue damage and persists long after the healing process has taken place, yet it is very difficult to tell when the organic pain ended and the psychogenic pain began (Fordyce, 1986). As with the other disorders in this group the absence of organic cause and unremitting persistence are diagnostic features.

Although it is understandable why somatoform pain disorder is in the classification its features need refinement and greater specificity before they can be regarded as satisfactory.

## DISSOCIATIVE DISORDERS

The concept of dissociation, or splitting, first described satisfactorily by the French psychiatrist, Pierre Janet (1894), is the essential feature of this group of disorders. The normal integration of emotion, sensation, movement and thinking is impaired. However, this does not proceed to disintegration of these functions, as in schizophrenia, and compensation for the handicaps produced is often so good that the average external observer will notice nothing wrong.

When dissociation affects the highest level of organisation, the personality, the condition is described as multiple personality disorder, and other types of dissociation are classified according to the major functions affected, i.e. complex behaviour (fugues and possession states), movement (e.g. paralysis, stupor), memory (psychogenic amnesia), sensation, and perception (depersonalization) (Table 6.4).

The descriptions of all these disorders are qualified by additional statements referring to the common presence of psychological stressors immediately preceding the onset of the disorder and the absence of any physical disorder that could similarly explain the symptoms. This is because dissociative disorders are often crude imitations of well-known organic diseases; they are mimics rather than original actors, and their range of roles is remarkable. This is stony ground for the nosologist dependent on presenting features for description of disorder and it has not been an easy task to classify this group.

Table 6.4 Classification of dissociative disorders in DSM-III-R and ICD-10

| Type | DSM-III-R | ICD-10 |
|---|---|---|
| Dissociation of personality | Multiple Personality Disorder: 'existence within the person of two or more distinct personalities' and 'at least two of these personalities recurrently take full control of the person's behaviour | Multiple personality disorder: two or more distinct personalities with only one of them being evident at a time (included among 'other types of dissociative and conversion disorders', not as a separate category) |
| Dissociation of complex behaviours | Psychogenic Fugue: sudden unexpected travel away from home, with inability to recall one's past and the assumption of a new identity | Psychogenic fugue: 'an apparently purposeful journey away from home or place of work during which self-care is maintained' associated with the features of psychogenic amnesia |
| | | Trance and possession states: temporary loss of 'the sense of personal identity and full awareness of surroundings' |
| Dissociation of movement | Conversion Disorder: non-conscious impaired physical functioning suggesting a physical disorder when none is present, with aetiologically related psychological factors (included in the somatoform disorders) | Psychogenic stupor: 'a profound diminution or absence of voluntary movement and normal responsiveness to external stimuli such as light, noise and touch' |
| | | Psychogenic disorders of voluntary movement, and psychogenic convulsions |
| Dissociation of cognitive function | Psychogenic Amnesia: sudden inability 'to recall important personal information' that is too great or significant to be explained by forgetfulness | Psychogenic amnesia: amnesia (partial or complete) 'centred around traumatic events' that is 'not due to organic mental disorder, and is too great to be explained by ordinary forgetfulness or fatigue' |

Table 6.4 (*contd.*)

| Type | DSM-III-R | ICD-10 |
|------|-----------|--------|
| Dissociation of sensation | As for Conversion Disorder (see above) | Psychogenic anaesthesia and sensory loss: including complaints of paraesthesia (e.g. pins and needles), impaired vision, psychogenic deafness and loss of smell (anosmia) |
| Dissociation of perception | Depersonalization Disorder: persisting or recurrent depersonalization including (1) feeling detached from one's self 'as if one is an outside observer of one's mental processes or body', or (2) 'feeling like an automaton or as if in a dream'. This must be of sufficient severity to cause 'marked distress' yet 'intact reality testing is maintained | Depersonalization– Derealization syndrome: a spontaneous complaint that 'mental activity, body, and/or surroundings' are altered in quality. For a definite diagnosis the subject must have depersonalization symptoms (recognition that one's own experience is, or feelings are, odd or changed in some way) and/or derealisation symptoms (a similar feeling with regard to objects, people or surroundings), provided that these changes are accepted as subjective and spontaneous and not imposed by external forces, and present in a clear sensorium |
| Other types of dissociation | Ganser Syndrome, derealisation in the absence of depersonalisation, trance states | Transient amnesic or trance states often found in children and adolescence, Ganser syndrome |

## Dissociation of personality

This condition is the only specified personality disorder diagnosed as a mental disorder and has been described consistently since the first report in 1816 (Cutler and Reed, 1975). Although from the point of view of simple description this is illogical the rapidity and reversibility of the changes, which can involve up to 30 different personalities in the same individual at different times, separates it easily from typical personality disorders, which show enduring features from adolescence onwards, and from the ICD-10 diagnosis of 'personality change' which is often insidious and not a reversible process.

In clinical practice it is impossible to get away from the dynamic concept of secondary gain with multiple personalities; they serve a protective purpose and often follow a traumatic event, best exemplified by the famous case described by Thigpen and Cleckley (1954) (subsequently made into a popular film) in which the personality changes followed bereavement in a vulnerable young woman.

## Dissociation of complex behaviours

These include classical fugue and trance states which are perhaps the most familiar of all dissociative disorders. They show marked differences in incidence and presentation between cultures (Sargant, 1957) and are particularly related to major stress such as that found in post-traumatic stress disorder (Chapter 7). They are particularly common in wartime, when they often show a dramatic response to abreactive treatments (Grinker and Spiegel, 1943; Sargant and Shorvon, 1945).

There is little difficulty in making the diagnosis of a psychogenic fugue when all the elements are present although there is a suspicion in many clinician's minds that the behaviours carried out in a fugue state are so complex that some at least must be carried out in full consciousness and could therefore be regarded as malingering. There is also some overlap with multiple personality disorder (Cutler and Reed, 1975). Psychogenic amnesia is an invariable component of the syndrome.

## Dissociation of movement or sensation

Classical 'conversion hysteria' associated with apparent muscular paralysis or equivalent sensory loss such as blindness is the core feature of this condition. Although the typical case is easy to identify in most instances, it can present many problems in others, supporting Slater's (1965) view that the diagnosis of hysteria is 'a fertile ground for clinical error'. Merskey (1986) cites paroxysmal hemicrania, thoracic outlet syndrome, spastic oesophagus, facial dyskinesia, torticollis, painful leg/moving toes and the whiplash syndrome as conditions that are commonly diagnosed as conversion phenomena. The same difficulties are even more apparent with epilepsy (Fenton, 1986) and with hysterical stupor, in which the absence of movement and verbal contact deprives the psychiatrist of his main sources of information, and still leads to misdiagnosis of encephalitis and other brain disease particularly when it involves the midbrain.

Although the original descriptions of conversion hysteria emphasised the equanimity of the patient in the face of a major handicap (e.g. Charcot, 1889; Janet, 1984) *la belle indifférence* (as it was called) is not now considered to be particularly important in making the diagnosis. Psychophysiological studies of these patients, ever since the original study of Lader and Sartorious (1968), have persistently found that they are hyperaroused (e.g. Mears and Horvath, 1972).

Although this disorder has to be classified under somatoform disorders in DSM-III-R because of its primary somatic presentation, it is uneasy in this company. In most cases there is a clear psychosocial stressor and the nature of the symptom (e.g. writer's cramp) is often linked closely to the nature of the stress. This does not apply to other somatoform disorders. As these associations are part of dynamic interpretation that is so loathed by current nosologists, the difficulties do not intrude into the written descriptions but they are none the less present as the hidden agenda of diagnosis.

## Dissociation of cognitive function

Psychogenic amnesia is such a common component of dissociative disorders that it could be regarded as a redundant diagnosis. It is certainly at a lower level in the hierarchy of dissociation than both fugue states and multiple personality and is an essential element of both of these. However, there are other instances, of which Mr Brown described earlier (case history 6.2) is a good example, where psychogenic amnesia is the predominant feature and therefore constitutes the main diagnosis.

Amnesia is also impossible to differentiate into dissociative or conscious types and the only useful aid is the concept of unconscious motivation. Does the amnesia make clinical sense when taken in conjunction with its antecedents and present setting? If the 'fit' is poor, alternatives need to be sought and even if the diagnosis of psychogenic amnesia is chosen the possibility of malingering will never be far away.

## Dissociation of perception

Depersonalisation is the main member of this set of conditions. It is an unusual symptom that is known to be part of phobic (Roth, 1959) and generalized anxiety (Fewtrell, 1984), depressive illness and schizophrenia as well as a primary syndrome (Ackner, 1959). In ICD-9 it was described as:

> an unpleasant state of disturbed perception in which external objects or parts of one's own body are experienced as changed in their quality, unreal, remote or automatized. The patient is aware of the subjective nature of the change he experiences.

The essential elements of this description are maintained in ICD-10 (Table 6.4), but in DSM-III-R the diagnosis of depersonalization disorder is confined to depersonalization experiences alone. The reasoning behind this division is not clear, and in European psychiatry the differences between depersonalization (altered perception of self) and derealization (altered perception of surroundings) have never been regarded as of diagnostic significance.

Depersonalization looks a little out of place amongst the other dissociative disorders. Disturbances in identity, memory or consciousness are said by DSM-III-R to be the essential features of the dissociative group, and depersonalization is none of these. It is a state of altered perception in almost pure form and although in DSM-III-R its inclusion is defended on the grounds of identity disturbance this appears somewhat specious. It is rather less of an identity disturbance than borderline personality disorder or transexualism and certainly has none of the cognitive splitting that is the foundation of dissociation. In previous classifications depersonalization was included amongst the neuroses; if the term had not been abolished it would still be there.

## Other types of dissociation

These include trance and possession states, evocatively described in William Sargant's *Battle for the Mind* (1957), dissociative states of short duration in adolescents and young adults (sometimes collectively included under the heading of epidemic hysteria (Merskey, 1979, p. 174), and hysterical pseudodementia or the Ganser syndrome.

Of these the Ganser syndrome has aroused the most interest for nosology. It was first described in three prisoners awaiting trial (Ganser, 1898) who in their responses to questioning showed the essential feature of *Vorbeireden*, a German word which is difficult to translate but which includes the element of skirting round a subject closely. This has led to the Ganser syndrome being described as the syndrome of approximate answers', as questions are answered wrongly but are so close to being correct that the questioner suspects the correct answer is known. If 'five' is the response to 'How many legs has a cow?' ignorance could just about be suspected, but when '99' is given as the answer to 'What are 50 plus 50?' the rules of chance association are stretched.

In Ganser's original description there were disturbances of consciousness, the hysterical 'twilight state', as well as hallucinations and conversion symptoms. The true Ganser syndrome is rare and should certainly be included amongst the dissociative states, but Ganser symptoms are common in a wide range of psychiatric disorders, including depression and schizophrenia, as well as in organic brain disease (Whitlock, 1967) and in such cases should be classified with the primary pathology.

## Summary

In summary, the dissociative disorders are a mixture of conditions, many of which are uncommon and getting more so, that are held together by only a few common threads. Their classification by description only is fraught with error because they are so intimately related to the stresses that precipitated them and the social setting in which the symptoms are expressed (Mayou, 1976). As they have been such a fecund source of hypotheses about mental illness their relegation to an atheoretical system of classification has stultified rather than enlightened their status.

# ANALYSIS

## Clarity

At one level the somatoform and dissociative disorders are clear and unambiguous. Because the main features of the disorders are focused as bodily complaints or specific loss of function they are easily identifiable. For example, the disturbance of a psychogenic fugue and the complaints in somatoform pain disorder are so distinctive that it would be extremely difficult to misidentify the symptoms. In the case of the somatoform disorders the symptoms can be linked readily to the appropriate functional system, and the persistence of these symptoms with the refusal to accept medical reassurance are only too obvious from the history. In fact, the psychiatrist is likely to be reminded of these features repeatedly in the course of interviewing a typical patient without having to look specifically for any of the diagnostic criteria. The problem with these disorders is not detection but interpretation. Are the symptoms consciously induced, in which case they can only be described as malingering, even though this is seldom a full explanation of the problem since most malingerers have other psychiatric abnormality (Flicker, 1956), or are the symptoms unconscious in origin and the victim blameless of any wish to deceive? The question is impossible to answer.

There is another difficulty in the interpretation of bodily symptoms. Almost all people present to doctors with bodily complaints of varying degrees of severity and persistence. Their evaluation is the main reason why medical students need at least five years of training before they are considered competent. Weighing the significance of symptoms and observation is extremely difficult and is one of the reasons why medicine is still regarded as an art rather than a science in many quarters.

A satisfactory diagnosis is one that is based on a set of features that leads the investigator on a road which only has one destination. The complaints of feeling the cold persistently, getting exhausted after little effort, and putting on weight are shared by thousands of individuals, but if the clinician suspects myxodoema because of additional evidence on examination (e.g. slow pulse rate, delayed tendon reflexes), and subsequently finds thyroxine deficiency on laboratory examination, the diagnosis is confirmed without any degree of doubt. The problem with diagnosing the somatoform and dissociative disorders is that the investigator receives no positive diagnostic information beyond the first stage of diagnosis, the presentation the symptom. Throughout the descriptions of these disorders in DSM-III-R and ICD-10 there are reminders that physical disorders must be excluded before the mental diagnosis can be made. This throws a great deal of responsibility on to the psychiatrist because the assumption is made that he or she, together with other medical colleagues, can exclude organic disease with a high degree of confidence. The neurologist, Henry Miller, who was also trained in psychiatry, once commented that an ordinary doctor needed to be a reasonably competent physician but a psychiatrist needed to be a superlative one, as he or she had to know the full range of manifestations of physical disease before making any psychiatric diagnosis (Miller, 1987).

The reality is that no doctor can be absolutely confident of excluding physical disorder and this is acknowledged implicitly in the wording of both formal classifications. Thus in DSM-III-R the door is left open for the possibility that somatoform disorders may have an, as yet unknown, physical cause by the statement 'although the symptoms of somatoform disorders are "physical", the specific pathophysiologic processes involved are not demonstrable or understandable by existing laboratory procedures', and the diagnosis of the dissociative disorder in ICD-10 'should remain probable or provisional if there is any doubt about the contribution of existing or possible physical disorders, or if it is impossible to achieve an understanding of why the disorder has developed'.

Nevertheless, despite these criticisms, the diagnosis of the different somatoform and dissociative disorders is reasonably clear provided that one accepts that all reasonable attempts to make an organic diagnosis have been made and the possibility excluded.

## Overlap

Consideration will first be given to the overlap between the somatoform and dissociative disorders themselves and then attention will be turned to the three groups of conditions that overlap continually with them: affective states, multi-system physical diseases, and personality disorders.

### Overlap between Somatoform and Dissociative Disorders

Such differences that there are between the ICD-10 and DSM-III-R classifications reflect a difference of emphasis, with the American classification giving much greater precedence to the somatoform group, which in statistical terms is much larger. Although the two classifications differ little in their handling of dissociative disorders by using the simple device of classifying them according to the function affected, which is preferable to the older terminology based on the organs concerned (e.g. globus hystericus, hysterical paraplegia), there is dispute about what should be included in the dissociative group. Thus classical conversion disorder with physical symptoms is classified with the somatoform group in DSM-III-R whereas in ICD-10 it is one of the core groups of dissociative disorder with various subclassifications. DSM-III-R illustrates the debt it owes to Guze and his group in demolishing hysteria as a diagnostic term by including conversion hysteria as a somatoform disorder. This seems illogical as conversion hysteria in DSM-III-R is the only somatoform disorder that allows dynamic mechanisms to enter into the formation of the diagnosis, so that the symptoms are 'apparently an expression of a psychological conflict or need', which in any case abandons Guze's original premise, that 'the term conversion symptom carries with it no etiological pathogenic implications' (Guze, 1970). DSM-III-R also allows a simultaneous presence of another classical tenet of hysteria, *la belle indifférence*, although it comments that the symptom is of little diagnostic value.

There is also some argument over the status of depersonalization. This is given greater diagnostic weight than derealization in DSM-III-R and is included as a dissociative disorder whereas in ICD-10 it has its own diagnostic category within the neurotic disorders. DSM-III-R stresses that the depersonalization experience must be associated with marked distress whereas this is not necessary in ICD-10. Both classifications emphasise that depersonalization is a symptom that occurs in the presence of panic, obsessive–compulsive neurosis, depression and schizophrenic disorders and in any of these conditions it should be regarded as a secondary phenomenon. Nevertheless, there are occasions when depersonalization appears to be the primary experience and other symptoms are secondary to this. The feeling of being cut off from reality and acting like an automaton can be extremely unpleasant and patients often describe the chronology of such disorders as beginning with a state of depersonalization.

The other dissociative disorders are largely self-explanatory and it is difficult to see how they could be misclassified or confused where they present in typical form. Multiple personality disorder is a rare but well-described condition made famous by the case studies of Morton Prince (1905) and by several movie films, the most noted of which is *The Three Faces of Eve*. Psychogenic fugues and amnesias have long been recognised as rare but distinctive reactions to tremendous stress, with a higher incidence in wartime (Grinker and Spiegel, 1943). Psychogenic amnesia is a common accompaniment to fugues and multiple personality disorder and its convenient presence at times when knowledge would expose the fiction of the disorder is often important diagnostically.

There is more certainty in the somatoform disorders. Although the concept of unconscious motivation has been abandoned by DSM-III-R it remains waiting in the shadows in classifying all disorders in this group. In general, although it is an oversimplification, the disorders in which there is a close and understandable link between stressor and symptoms tend to be classified as dissociative whereas if such links are few or absent and the complaint is of bodily symptoms the diagnosis becomes that of a somatoform disorder.

There is considerable difficulty in separating hypochondriasis and somatization disorders because their symptomatology may be identical. In making the distinction between them ICD-10 gives useful guidelines which make good clinical sense. 'In somatization disorders, the emphasis is on the symptoms themselves and their individual effects, whereas in hypochondriasis attention is directed more to the presence of an underlying progressive and serious disease process that has disabling consequences. In hypochondriasis the patient tends to ask for investigations to determine or confirm the nature of the underlying disease, whereas the patient with somatization disorder asks for treatment to remove the symptoms.' In the age of the consumer it is only right that consumerism should have a say in diagnosis.

## Overlap with Affective States

Somatization is a well-established accompaniment of affective states, notably depressive illness (Lewis, 1934) and the somatic symptoms of anxiety can also be expressed as a primary complaint (Tyrer, 1976). Indeed, when patients with a DSM-III diagnosis of agoraphobia with panic were formally tested for the presence of DSM-III somatization disorder using an interview schedule, 27% (12 out of 44) met the stringent criteria for somatization disorder compared with none from a control group (King *et al.*, 1986). It is also common for depression and anxiety to accompany somatoform and dissociative disorders except when classical *belle indifférence* is present. It is often extremely difficult for the clinician to decide which condition is primary and, because depression and anxiety are generally easier to treat than somatoform and dissociative disorders, the affective diagnosis tends to be made more readily and treated accordingly. The early onset of classical somatization disorder will also exclude those patients who present with somatic symptoms after the age of 35 where the affective diagnosis is more likely. However, the case of Mrs Mackie (case history 6.1) demonstrates that this distinction is far from clear-cut and perhaps the diagnosis of an affective disorder, particularly depressive illness, is made too readily.

## Overlap with Multisystem Physical Diseases

The problem in differentiating somatization and dissociation disorders from physical illness has already been mentioned. The diagnosis of any of these disorders can seldom be unequivocal and in some ways it is sad to report that one of the firmest guides to the diagnosis is the history of a previous episode (Cloninger, 1987). Put another way, the fact that there has been a similar condition in the past *not* followed by a physical disease gives more diagnostic reassurance than any number of operational criteria. The multi-system involvement of symptoms in somatization disorder might appear to carry diagnostic weight, but as systematic lupus erythematosus and other autoimmune disorders, intermittent acute porphyria and other rare metabolic diseases, and electrolyte disturbance can all lead to symptoms in many organs, their clinical picture can be identical to that in somatization disorder. They should all be considered before the diagnosis of any of the somatoform disorders is made. Every clinician who is involved in the successful diagnosis of these disorders will be aware of the many psychiatric misdiagnoses, often expressed in terms of 'functional overlay' or 'hysterical elaboration', that are commonplace before the underlying disorder is recognised. The operational criteria of DSM-III-R are no protection: most of these multisystem diseases can satisfy all of them without difficulty.

Despite this problem there are subtle differences between these symptomatically identical physical and psychiatric disorders. Often these are recognised at an intuitive level only; something suspicious about the presentation of the disorder impels the clinician to carry out further physical investigations and laboratory tests until the correct diagnosis is discovered. The condition looks 'as if' it is a psychiatric disorder but there is something suspicious about it: its suddenness of onset, its clean separation from all previous functioning, or its complete lack of association with environmental stimuli. This clinical 'sixth sense' needs to be trained and better formalised because it is invaluable. When it is absent the alternatives of missing physical diagnoses or of reinforcing somatoform ones by unnecessary tests are prejudicial to both competence and reputation.

In clinical practice, however, it is at least as common to find 'hysterical' symptomatology in settings where organic disease is widespread, and psychiatric and physical disorders often coexist. There is a much higher representation of conversion disorders in neurological settings than psychiatric ones (Whitlock, 1967; Merskey and Buhrich, 1975) and separating one from the other requires some luck as well as clinical finesse.

## Overlap with Personality Disorders

The association between somatoform and dissociative disorders and personality disturbance, particularly of a histrionic nature, has attracted attention repeatedly. The assumption is made in these enquiries that two conditions, an Axis I and an Axis II disorder, are present simultaneously. An alternative explanation is that the personality disturbance is the only disorder and its manifestations include physical or other symptoms of insignificant status as mental disorder, a position acknowledged to some extent by the diagnosis of factitious disorder in DSM-III-R

The distinction from personality disorder is made more difficult by the chronic nature of many of the somatoform group disorders. When symptoms, and their associated patterns of behaviour, have been present for most of the person's adult life, it is difficult not to regard them as intrinsic to the personality. There are two major types of personality disturbance associated with somatization. The first is included within the flamboyant group of DSM-III personality disorders (Frances, 1980) and includes histrionic and antisocial personality disorders. There is a great deal of evidence showing association between the 'hysterical' group of disorders and this type of personality disturbance (Cloninger and Guze, 1970; Guze *et al.*, 1971a; Cloninger *et al.*, 1975; Guze *et al.*, 1986). In general these studies show that conversion symptomatology is more common with these personality disorders although there have been criticisms of the descriptions of this symptomatology which shows a very large female to male sex ratio (Guze *et al.*, 1972). The other group of disorders is included within the inhibited, fearful group (Frances, 1980; Ferguson and Tyrer, 1988). Indeed, within this group we have found good evidence for the existence of hypochondriacal personality disorder as a separate subtype (Tyrer and Alexander, 1988). In addition to hypochondriacal personality traits, this group has high ratings for anxiousness and conscientiousness and is quite different from the histrionic and sociopathic personality disorders. When such patterns of thinking and behaviour have persisted throughout adult life it is more reasonable to regard them as part of a personality disturbance rather than a neurotic syndrome and, the 'double diagnosis' of hypochondriacal neurosis and personality disorder is not of much value.

## Outcome

One of the strongest arguments justifying the introduction of somatization disorder (and its precursor, Briquet's syndrome) to diagnostic practice was the evidence of its consistency over time (Guze, 1970). We now have a long period of follow-up, up to 12 years, of patients originally diagnosed with Briquet's syndrome by Guze and his colleagues at Washington University School of Medicine in St Louis. Unlike in many follow-up studies, assessments were made blind to the original diagnosis (Martin *et al.*, 1979) and showed that most patients diagnosed with definite or probable Briquet's syndrome (23 out of 36) still had the same diagnosis 6–12 years later (Guze *et al.*, 1986).

This level of consistency is not shown by the dissociative group of disorders. Indeed, the absence of consistency was one of the reasons why Eliot Slater (1965) suggested that the diagnosis of hysteria should be abandoned and the word used only in its adjectival form.

He based his conclusion largely on a nine-year follow-up study of 85 patients given a firm diagnosis of hysteria. Of these no less than 46 were found to have organic disease at follow-up, half of whom developed their disease in the follow-up period (so by implication the 'hysteria' was likely to be a prodrome or early stage of the illness). Another ten developed schizophrenia or affective psychosis and 14 developed what would now be described as somatization disorder with multiple somatic symptoms and personality disturbance. Only seven retained the original diagnosis of hysteria with classical conversion symptoms. However, it is important to realise that Slater's population was seen in a specialised hospital for neurological disorders. Other studies (Lewis, 1975; Reed, 1975) have shown that organic illness is much less common at follow-up and there is still a small nucleus of between 10% and 15% of patients who retain the diagnosis of primary hysterical disorder. When the hysterical symptoms are found in conjunction with, or are extremely difficult to separate from, another physical condition the persistence is greater. A classical example is hystero-epilepsy. It is extremely difficult to disentangle hystero-epilepsy from true epilepsy (Fenton, 1986), and the outcome of hystero-epilepsy, with a pattern of behaviour persisting for many years, does not show the same diagnostic shifts as other conversion of dissociative reactions. Again, however, it is extremely difficult to be certain in the cases in which the apparent hysterical symptoms persist that these are not secondary to underlying true epileptic disturbance.

It therefore appears that only about 10% of dissociative states persist and if cases of 'epidemic hysteria' are taken into account the proportion is even less. When hysteria occurs in epidemic form it is often associated with a powerful event or individual and the effects are greater if the victims are impressionable and part of the same organisation or group. Under these circumstances it is perhaps not surprising that many epidemics are described in girls' boarding schools (e.g. Moss and McEvedy, 1966; Benaim *et al.*, 1973). It is important to add that there are many other examples in which epidemics occur in other settings and that gender is relatively unimportant. The outcome of this type of hysteria is almost uniformly good although no adequate long-term follow-up has been reported.

## Treatment

The treatment of dissociative and somatoform disorders is not particularly helpful with regard to classification. This is because there is no satisfactory treatment for either group of conditions. Early intervention from the psychiatric services may be extremely valuable and a single interview followed by advice for general practitioners and other primary care workers can be extremely effective in reducing subsequent morbidity (e.g. Smith *et al.*, 1986). Various forms of hypnotherapy and psychotherapy have been recommended for hysterical states and were present at the dawn of psychoanalysis when Freud and Breuer first became involved in the psychotherapy of hysterical states. Despite much interest there have been no satisfactory studies of the various forms of treatment ranging from hypnotherapy through to behavioural forms of management and in view of the evanescent nature of many hysterical states anecdotal reports of successful treatment are of little value.

CHAPTER 7

# Stress and Adjustment Disorders

These conditions are characterised by the close relationship between a clear-cut external stressor and both the onset and maintenance of the disorder. In addition, the manifestations of the disorder
include mood and behaviour disturbance. Both these are extremely
variable in form and persistence but their content often has links
with the precipitating stressor. In many respects the conditions
have been the forgotten majority of psychiatriac disorders although
recently they have attracted more attention. In particular, post-
traumatic stress disorder has had a high profile in the United States
since the Vietnam War with considerable research carried out into
the criteria necessary for making the diagnosis. One stimulus for
this has been the medico-legal implications of this particular
diagnosis.

   There are very few differences between the two major classifications in their description of adjustment and stress disorders although in practice there is some difficulty in making firm diagnoses
and there have been no satisfactory studies of their reliability.
However, typical examples of each of the disorders are readily
identified as can be gathered by the following descriptions.

## Case histories

### 7.1   Acute Stress Reaction

Miss Doolittle was 25 and engaged to be married. Four days before the wedding her fiancé phoned her up to tell her he was not going through with the marriage. After hearing this news she became extremely distressed and was almost incoherent when she visited her parents nearby a few minutes later. She kept on repeating her fiancé's name but would not explain what had happened. She was taken to a casualty department but by the time she was seen by the casualty officer she had collected herself and was able to give a good account of the problem. She was unable to explain adequately her feelings after hearing the telephone call and expressed strong feelings of anger as well as other emotions towards her boyfriend. The next day she was completely recovered and, although still upset at the thought of the break-up, took the major part in informing the wedding guests that the marriage would not now take place.

## 7.2   Adjustment Disorder

Mr Farrell was 25 and had always had difficulty in making relationships. He had been in care for five years as a child and had never known his father. After leaving school he had a series of jobs, all unskilled, none of which lasted for longer than six months. Although he had no difficulty in developing relationships with girls he found it very difficult to maintain these because of his unpredictability and unstable lifestyle. However, just before his twenty-fourth birthday he met a girl with whom he developed his first close relationship and they decided to live together soon afterwards. He got a regular job as a warehouseman and all seemed to be going well. Unfortunately he returned home one evening to find that his girlfriend had gone and she had left a note saying that she had returned to live with her parents in another town. He spent the next few days trying to contact her without success and when eventually he found out where she was living she refused to speak to him. He told her parents that if she would not talk to him he would kill himself. Subsequently he took an overdose of paracetamol and was admitted to a psychiatric unit after expressing continuing suicidal feelings at assessment.

He recovered rapidly in hospital and lost his suicidal feelings almost immediately. He showed no evidence of depressive symptomatology but said that he could not stop thinking about his girlfriend and how badly she had treated him. He was discharged from hospital after four days and when seen three weeks later as an outpatient had already developed a relationship with a new girlfriend. Nevertheless, he continued to remain bitter about his past relationship and was extremely angry when his former girlfriend's name was mentioned.

## 7.3   Post-traumatic Stress Disorder

Mr Boot was a lorry driver who had never had an accident in 20 years of driving. One day while driving on a country road he was unable to stop when a van pulled out in front of him. His recollection of what happened next was poor and he could only recall staggering out of his cab and walking towards the other vehicle, where he saw a man lying across the seat motionless with blood all over his face. At first he thought the man was dead but although the other driver had sustained a broken leg he made a full recovery later.

Although Mr Boot appeared to make a good recovery from this experience he started to have difficulty in sleeping some two weeks after the accident. He had nightmares of driving in the dark and having collisions, after which he woke in a sweat. Shortly afterwards he could not stop thinking about the face of the injured man and described it as 'like a shadow in the back of my mind'. He was referred to an outpatient clinic and treated with cognitive therapy and anxiety management. He showed some improvement with this and was able to return to work shortly afterwards. However, he was unable to travel on long journeys and often became extremely anxious when driving on open roads. Although he continued to improve one year after the accident he was still reluctant to travel long distances and refused to go on the route where the accident had occurred. By this time he had no other symptoms. Twenty-two months after the accident he came in triumph to his regular outpatient appointment to say that he had just completed the first journey over the same route as the accident without any problems. He remained free of symptoms and showed no avoidance of any situation after this time.

There is little difficulty in distinguishing between the conditions exemplified by these three case histories. The first is typical of what is perceived by the lay public as acute stress, with the break-up of an engagement, a major unexpected even of great personal significance, occurring just before marriage, at a time when emotions tend to be heightened. Under these circumstances it was almost normal to have great difficulty in adjusting to the stress at first. The symptoms of behaviour shown by Miss Doolittle probably represent a composite mixture of emotions, including anger with her boyfriend, humiliation in front of her friends and relatives, anxiety about the immediate future and depression about the loss of the engagement. It is very difficult to cope with all these emotions simultaneously and present an appropriate exterior to the world. However, in an acute stress reaction there is rapid adjustment to the stress and within a few hours Miss Doolittle was able to face herself and the world again.

Mr Farrell (case history 7.2) has a more complex problem. He already has many problems in his life and, not surprisingly, has invested a great deal in his relationship with his first steady girlfriend. When she leaves him he is devastated but does not have the emotional resources to adjust to this. The overdose taken because his girlfriend refused to speak to him is an all too familiar pattern of emotional blackmail found in these situations. Although he had serious depressive symptoms they were only present for a short time and the almost complete resolution of these when he was admitted to hospital is also characteristic of adjustment disorders. His subsequent improvement and involvement with a new girlfriend illustrates the speed at which his affections could change although his continued bitterness about the loss showed that this adjustment was by no means complete.

Mr Boot's problem (case history 7.3) is representative of post-traumatic stress disorder and satisfies all the diagnostic criteria for the condition. Although car accidents are all too common those that are associated with major injury are much less so and the events of his accident are outside the realm of normal stressful experience. The most harrowing part of this was seeing the other driver covered with blood and apparently dead. The delay before the onset of insomnia and other symptoms, the persistently intrusive image of the injured man, and his increased anxiety and reluctance to drive on open road again are all characteristic of post-traumatic stress disorder. In Mr Boot's case he responded well to cognitive 'restructuring' of the accident and his reaction to it and was also helped significantly by anxiety management and relaxation. Nevertheless, he took nearly two years to shake off the symptoms and the condition entirely. Unfortunately some patients with post-traumatic stress disorder do not make a full recovery and are left with chronic disability.

The separation of these three groups of disorder in DSM-III-R and ICD-10 is reasonably clear-cut (Table 7.1) and, in the case of post-traumatic stress disorder, very specific (Table 7.2). The different time course is immediately apparent, with acute reactions lasting only a few days compared with up to six months for adjustment disorder and even longer periods for post-traumatic stress disorder. The adjustment disorders are further subdivided into five or more categories depending on the primary manifestation of the disorder: anxiety or depressive symptoms, physical complaints, behaviour disturbance, or mixtures of these.

Post-traumatic stress disorder is the best-researched condition in this group. Although its main features have, been recognised for many years (e.g. Daly, 1983; Jablensky, 1985) it only became formalised in psychiatric terms during the Second World War, particularly by Kardiner (1941). It had to wait until 1978 before there was (hard-won) agreement for it to be included as a diagnosis among the neurotic disorders following many prominent examples of the condition during the war in Vietnam (Figley, 1978).

It still arouses controversy and there is considerable argument about its prevalence in people subjected to severe stress. These figures (summarised by Barlow, 1988, pp. 501–4) vary between 0% and 70%, and no satisfactory explanation for this is forthcoming.

Table 7.1 Classification of stress and adjustment disorders in DSM-III-R and ICD-10

| Diagnosis | DSM-III-R | ICD-10 |
|---|---|---|
| Acute Stress Reaction | Not included as a separate category in this classification | Transient disorder developing immediately in response to exceptional stress: diagnostic guidelines (i) mixed and changing picture of mood and behaviour, (ii) rapid resolution 'within a few hours at the most' if stress removed and within three days if stress not removed |
| Adjustment Disorder | A maladaptive reaction to an identifiable stressor which is not merely one instance of a pattern of over-reaction to a stressful circumstance. Diagnostic criteria: A maladaptive reaction as described above occurring within three months of onset of the stressor including either of the following: (1) impairment in occupational (including school) functioning or unusual social activities, (2) symptoms that are in excess of the normal and expectable [sic] reaction to the stressor(s). The reaction has lasted for no longer than six months and does not meet the criteria for any other mental disorder (including Uncomplicated Bereavement). Subclassified into adjustment disorder with: (a) Anxious mood (b) Depressed mood | States of distress and emotional disturbance 'arising in the period of adaptation to a significant life change or to the consequences of a stressful life event'. Diagnosis only made if (i) clear relationship between stressor and disturbance with onset within one month of stressful life event, with duration rarely exceeding six months, (ii) although individual vulnerability may predispose to occurrence 'the condition would not have arisen without the stressor'. May be classified according to subgroups: (a) brief depression reaction (less than one month), (b) prolonged depressive reaction (up to two years), (c) mixed anxiety and depressive reaction, (d) predominant disturbance of other emotions apart from depression, (e) predominant disturbance |

Table 7.1 (*contd.*)

| Diagnosis | DSM-III-R | ICD-10 |
|---|---|---|
| | (c) Disturbance of conduct <br> (d) Mixed disturbance of emotions and conduct <br> (e) Mixed emotional features <br> (f) Physical complaints <br> (g) With withdrawal <br> (h) With work and academic inhibition | of conduct (e.g. antisocial behaviour), (f) mixed disturbance of emotions and conduct |

The DSM-III-R requirements for the diagnosis include presence of the symptoms for at least one month; this can help in excluding disturbance of shorter duration that resolves spontaneously and could well be included under acute stress or adjustment disorders.

## ANALYSIS

### Clarity

The descriptions of the three main groups of stress and adjustment disorders are clear and have the advantage of being confined to a limited timescale. Acute stress disorder begins almost immediately after a major stress and resolves within a few days at the most, whereas adjustment disorders persist for much longer, particularly if the stressor giving rise to the disorder continues, although a time limit is set at six months. Post-traumatic stress disorder usually has a latent period of up to a month before the onset of symptoms (sometimes much longer, so that a delayed form of the condition is recognised with onset of symptoms six months or later after the trauma). The symptoms show a typical pattern, with intrusive reliving of the traumatic event coupled with its physical avoidance being associated with hyperarousal, usually in the form of anxiety.

It is of interest that symptoms in stress and adjustment disorders do not have the same status as in other psychiatric disorders. They do not dominate the classification process, so a mixture of emotions and/or behaviour disturbance is not only allowed but given formal status in the subclassification of adjustment disorders (Table 7.1). It

Table 7.2  Classification of Post-traumatic Stress Disorder in DSM-III-R and ICD-10

| DSM-III-R | ICD-10 |
|---|---|
| *Clinical description* | |
| The person has experienced an event that is outside the range of usual human experience and that would be markedly distressing to almost anyone, e.g. serious threat to one's life or physical integrity; serious threat or harm to one's children, spouse, or other close relatives and friends; sudden destruction of one's home or community; or seeing another person who has recently been or is being, seriously injured or killed as the result of an accident or physical violence | This arises as a delayed and/or protracted response to a stressful event or situation of an exceptionally threatening or catastrophic nature, which is likely to cause pervasive distress in almost anyone (e.g. natural or man-made disaster, combat, serious accident, witnessing the violent death of others, being the victim of torture, terrorism, rape, or other crime). If present, predisposing factors such as personality traits (e.g. compulsive, asthenic) or previous history or neurotic illness, may lower the threshold for the development of the syndrome or aggravate its course, but they are neither necessary nor sufficient to explain its occurrence. |
| | Typical features include episodes of repeated re-living of the trauma in intrusive memories ('flashbacks'), dreams or nightmares, occurring against the persisting background of a sense of 'numbness' and emotional blunting, detachment from other people, unresponsiveness to surroundings, anhedonia, and avoidance of activities and situations reminiscent of the trauma. Commonly there is fear and avoidance of cues reminding the sufferer of the original trauma. Rarely, there may be dramatic, acute bursts of fear, panic, or aggression, triggered by stimuli arousing a sudden recollection and/or re-enactment of the trauma or of the original reaction to it. There usually is a state of |

enhanced startle reaction, and insomnia. Anxiety and depression are commonly associated with the above symptoms and signs, and suicidal ideation is not infrequent. Drug or excessive alcohol use may be a complicating factor.

*Diagnostic guidelines*

This condition should not be diagnosed unless there is evidence that it had arisen within six months of a traumatic event of exceptional severity. A 'probable' diagnosis might still be possible if the delay between the event and the onset was longer than six months, provided that the clinical manifestations are typical and no alternative identification of the disorder (e.g. as an anxiety obsessive–compulsive, or depressive state) is plausible. In addition to evidence of trauma, there must be present a repetitive, intrusive recollection or re-enactment of the event in memories, daytime imagery, or dreams.

*(continued on p. 126)*

*Diagnostic criteria and guidelines*

The traumatic event is persistently reexperienced in at least one of the following ways:

(1) recurrent and intrusive distressing recollections of the event (in your children, repetitive play in which themes or aspects of the trauma are expressed)
(2) recurrent distressing dreams of the event
(3) sudden acting or feeling as if the traumatic event were recurring (include a sense of reliving the experience, illusions, hallucinations, and dissociative [flashback] episodes, even those that occur upon awakening or when intoxicated)
(4) intense psychological distress at exposure to events that symbolize or resemble an aspect of the traumatic event, including anniversaries of the trauma

Persistent avoidance of stimuli associated with the trauma or numbing of general responsiveness (not present before the trauma), as indicated by at least three of the following:

(1) efforts to avoid thoughts or feelings associated with the trauma
(2) efforts to avoid activities or situations that arouse recollections of the trauma

126

Table 7.2 (*contd.*)

| DSM-III-R | ICD-10 |
|---|---|
| (3) inability to recall an important aspect of the trauma (psychogenic amnesia)<br>(4) markedly diminished interest in significant activities (in young children, loss of recently acquired developmental skills such as toilet training or language skills)<br>(5) feeling of detachment or estrangement from others<br>(6) restricted range of affect, e.g., unable to have loving feelings<br>(7) sense of a foreshortened future, e.g., does not expect to have a career, marriage, or children, or a long life | A conspicuous emotional detachment, numbing of feeling, and avoidance of stimuli that might arouse recollection of the trauma are often present but are not essential for the diagnosis. |
| Persistent symptoms of increased arousal (not present before the trauma), as indicated by at least two of the following:<br><br>(1) difficulty falling or staying asleep<br>(2) irritability or outbursts of anger<br>(3) difficulty concentrating<br>(4) hypervigilance<br>(5) exaggerated startle response<br>(6) physiologic reactivity upon exposure to events that symbolize or resemble an aspect of the traumatic event (e.g., a woman who was raped in an elevator breaks out in a sweat when entering any elevator) | |
| Duration of the disturbance (symptoms in B, C, and D) of at least one month.<br><br>**Specify delayed onset** if the onset of symptoms was at least six months after the trauma. | The autonomic disturbances, mood disorder, and behavioural abnormalities are all contributory to the diagnosis but not of prime importance. |

s really the temporal connections rather than the symptoms themselves that are crucial in making the diagnosis.

One of the difficulties in making any of these diagnoses is that it is
impossible to predict the outcome if assessment is made at the
height of the episode, yet the likely outcome is a constituent of the
diagnosis. In practice the time course is probably retrospectively
assessed in most instances, the time of onset to the time of assessment being taken as the duration of the disorder. It is much easier to
reach a diagnosis at leisure some time after both the event and the
adjustment to it rather than in an emergency situation immediately
after the onset of symptoms.

The diagnosis of a stress and adjustment disorder is not made
when the symptoms persist long enough to qualify for another
neurotic diagnosis. Although this is an arbitrary decision it does
avoid confusion and aids the clarity of diagnosis.

Post-traumatic stress disorder is a clearly defined condition with
good reliability. Kappa values of inter-rater agreement were 0.85 in
one study (Blanchard *et al.*, 1986). This good agreement is partly to
be expected as both the symptoms and their precipitants are listed
clearly and contribute to the diagnosis. The traumatic event has to
be 'markedly distressing to almost anyone' in the words of DSM-III-
R. Such events include 'serious threat to one's life or physical
integrity; serious threat or harm to one's children, spouse or other
close relatives and friends; sudden destruction of one's home or
community; or seeing another person who has recently been, or is
being, seriously injured or killed as the result of an accident or
physical violence' (American Psychiatric Association, 1987, p. 250).
With this degree of specificity it can be seen readily that no other
diagnosis apart from post-traumatic stress disorder could be given
to Mr Boot's problem described above (case history 7.3).

## Overlap

There is little overlap between acute stress disorder and any other
psychiatric condition. The only possible exception is dissociative
disorders, which commonly begin immediately after a major stressful event but which demonstrate a more integrated and consistent
abnormality of symptoms or behaviour than do acute stress reactions. Thus the psychogenic fugue and amnesia are distinctive
abnormalities set in a context of otherwise normal function, whereas
the symptoms and behaviour at the height of an acute stress reaction
are essentially disintegrated; they represent the true meaning of
nervous breakdown.

Adjustment disorders merge into other neurotic diagnoses and in many cases this distinction is difficult to make. One is forced into making one diagnosis or the other on inadequate and subjective information about the time of onset of symptoms and value judgements made about the relative severity of different stressors. Curiously, once the threshold to another neurotic diagnosis has been crossed (e.g. the patient has four panic attacks) the nature of the stressor becomes unimportant in making the diagnosis. Although this is understandable it is none the less irritating to the clinician who would often like to have the stressor indicated in the diagnosis to differentiate it from similar symptom complexes that have no such precipitating circumstances.

Another difficulty, most commonly found with adjustment disorders, is in distinguishing the adjustment reaction from underlying personality disturbance. For example, although Mr Farrell's case (case history 7.2) is typical of an adjustment disorder, and almost certainly would not have come to psychiatric attention but for the stress created by his girlfriend leaving him, the rest of his history suggests a personality disorder, probably of the impulsive type (a new category in ICD-10 and DSM-III-R). As it is well established that the flamboyant group of personality disorders, including borderline, impulsive, narcissistic and histrionic personality disorders often react to adversity by extravagantly drawing attention to themselves and involving others in their problems (e.g. Chodoff and Lyons, 1958), the symptoms could be regarded as part of the disordered personality rather than a separate disorder of mental state. Transient, often severe, depression is frequent in borderline personality disorder (Gunderson and Singer, 1975; Gunderson and Elliott, 1985) and often occurs after stress.

There is some evidence that intrinsically these personality disorders create more adverse life events than those without abnormal personality (Seivewright, 1987, 1988) so adjustment reactions might be more common in personality-disordered individuals. This is supported by work showing a high incidence of abnormal personality (50%) in patients with adjustment disorder, 35% of whom had one of the flamboyant disorders described above (Tyrer *et al.*, 1988).

This difficulty is overcome to some extent by the stipulation in DSM-III-R that, to qualify for the diagnosis, the pattern of symptomatology and behaviour shown in an adjustment disorder must not be repetitive or recurrent. Thus Mr Farrell's overdose described in case history 7.2 could be regarded as an adjustment disorder if this was the first episode of this pattern of symptoms and behaviour. If similar episodes, not necessarily including an overdose, had been present in the past the diagnosis would not be entertained.

lthough this approach has merits it does severely reduce the
umbers receiving the diagnosis and poses the additional question
bout how the other group should be classified.

Post-traumatic stress disorder also shows little overlap with other
onditions, mainly because of its defined precipitants, although as it
ends to be persistent it may often be associated with other depres-
ive and anxiety disorders. The emotional numbness that is often
ound in the condition may also lead to some confusion with
lissociative disorders. The recurrent and unwelcome intrusion of
houghts about the traumatic event invites comparison with obses-
ional symptoms, and the avoidance of situations reminiscent of the
vent may be confused with phobic avoidance. In general, however,
he clear criteria for making the diagnosis are usually enough to
prevent significant overlap.

Both adjustment and post-traumatic stress disorders are de-
cribed in ICD-10 and DSM-III-R as occurring more often in those of
ulnerable personality. This implies that a lower level of stress is
equired to precipitate the disorder in vulnerable than in normal
ndividuals (Davidson *et al.*, 1985). Although this hypothesis has
eceived some support in one study (McKeon *et al.*, 1984) it is at
ariance with the alternative hypothesis that some personalities
create' more life events than others by their pattern of behaviour.
Comparison of life events and personality in adjustment and post-
raumatic stress disorders might offer an opportunity to test these
wo hypotheses. Personality status is at least as important in this
group of disorders as in other neurotic conditions where the associa-
ion with personality has long been recognised. It has particular
ignificance for studies of life events, as 'failure to take account of
he confounding variable of personality in investigations of life
vents before illness may produce misleading results in which the
ttachment of aetiological significance to events may be unjustified'
Seivewright, 1988, p. 92).

## Outcome

As mentioned earlier, the outcome of these disorders is incorporated into the diagnostic criteria. Stress and adjustment disorders
should resolve more or less entirely whereas post-traumatic stress
disorder may leave chronic residual disability. It would be extremely
useful to have some data on the outcome of conditions formally
classified as adjustment or stress disorders but little is available
apart from anecdotal reports.

One possible outcome is alcohol or drug abuse (Green *et al.*, 1983)
and this perhaps is understandable in view of the fact that many

sufferers from post-traumatic stress disorder are young men who may often turn to these ways of dealing with stress. This again raises the query of personality disorder in such instances. Are those with personality vulnerability more likely to suffer from post-traumatic as well as adjustment disorders and does this play the major part in outcome? I suspect that our findings with adjustment disorders are just as applicable to post-traumatic stress disorder. As it is much more 'respectable' to suffer from post-traumatic stress than personality disorder, the one is likely to be emphasised at the expense of the other, so it will not be easy to determine.

## Treatment

There are no clear-cut indications for treatment for any of these disorders. Both stress and adjustment disorders are, by definition, of short duration and implicitly carry the notion that resolution is possible without external intervention. However, it is generally accepted that this process can be facilitated by acceptance in full consciousness of the changes engendered by the stress. This process, often termed 'working through' the stressful experience and its effects, is well illustrated by Lindemann's (1944) classic paper on the Coconut Grove fire. By close follow-up of individuals involved in a major fire Lindemann was able to identify the characteristics that determined mental health outcome. Acceptance of unpleasant and often terrible personal experiences is distressing but it helps to promote successful adjustment. More significantly, it prevents the pathological consequences that ensue if adjustment is arrested or distorted. Lindemann's general findings have been confirmed in many subsequent studies (e.g. Kinston and Rosser, 1974; Green et al., 1983; Kilpatrick et al., 1985) and have promoted the development of psychotherapeutic interventions, both individual and group, in these disorders.

As the behavioural consequences of post-traumatic stress disorder include elements of both phobic avoidance and obsessional thoughts it is predictable that exposure therapies should be used in its management. However, these have not been used systematically in the same way as in phobic and obsessional disorders and the results are difficult to interpret. Nevertheless, exposure has become an established part of the psychotherapy of post-traumatic stress disorder and appears to be effective (Kuch et al., 1985; Horowitz, 1986).

There is surprisingly little information about the relative merits of drug and psychological treatments in stress and adjustment dis-

rders and there have been no satisfactory trials of drug interven-
ion (Van der Kolk, 1987). In general it is probably wise to avoid drug
reatment in these conditions except as emergency first-aid mea-
ures to control the stress when it is extreme (e.g. immediately after
he traumatic experience). There is an important caveat to this
dvice. In those instances where it is important for the patient to
vork through the exprience following the stress, drug therapy may
e counter-productive. For example, as it is well established that
enzodiazepines can create anterograde amnesia (Dundee and Pan-
lit, 1972) and other minor degees of memory disturbance they could
romote the mental mechanism of denial in adjustment and stress
lisorders if prescribed for any length of time. For this reason regular
reatment with these drugs in adjustment disorders should be
voided (Tyrer, 1989).

## SUMMARY

n summary, stress and adjustment disorders are reasonably well-
established diagnostic categories that are necessary in clinical prac-
ice. Post-traumatic stress disorder is better defined and described
nd, despite its late arrival on the diagnostic scene, has greater
alidity and reliability than the others in this group. Studies of their
egree of overlap, comparative outcome and response to treatment
re few but in general tend to support the distinction between the
hree disorders. The position of acute stress disorders is the least
atisfactory; its time course is so short that the argument for remov-
ng it from formal diagnosis is a strong one.

CHAPTER 8

# General Neurotic Syndrome and Mixed Anxiety–Depressive Disorders

Previous chapters have been concerned primarily with comparing the two standard classifications of neurotic disorder and examining the validity for the distinction between different conditions. This chapter is different: it introduces a new concept, the 'general neurotic syndrome', which is not part of any existing classification. It postulates the existence of a mixed neurotic syndrome in which symptoms of anxiety and depression predominate but which can also have elements of other neurotic disorder at any time. Its description may appear to be retrograde in a classificatory sense, harking back to the beginning of this century when it was suggested that there were two chief functional disorders, one of neurosis and the other psychosis (the *Einheitneurosen* and *Einheitpsychosen* of the German school). The diagnosis of general neurotic syndrome does not, however, exclude the individual diagnostic disorders described in other parts of this book, although if any condition always satisfies the criteria for a mixed syndrome it would have little justification for being separately named. The introduction of the syndrome is a plea for acceptance of mixed syndromes in formal classification of neurotic disorder in the same way that mixed symptoms are allowed for other conditions in both ICD-10 and DSM-III-R classifications.

Table 8.1   Causes of difficulty in diagnosis of neurotic disorders in DSM-
III-R and ICD-10

| Characteristic | Deficiency |
|---|---|
| Symptoms and diagnosis | High co-morbidity |
| Stability | Frequent change in diagnosis over time |
| Time course | Necessity for different durations of symptoms for different diagnoses |
| Treatment response | Similar response to treatment in main diagnoses apart from phobic and obsessional disorders |
| Personality status | Frequently occurs with neurotic disorders but is not considered in making the diagnosis |

## DEFICIENCIES OF CURRENT CLASSIFICATION

The main deficiencies of ICD-10 and DSM-III-R classification of
neurotic disorder are illustrated in Table 8.1. It is worthwhile
discussing these separately because they are all used at different
times by those who reject the idea of diagnosis entirely in this group
of disorders.

### Individual symptoms and diagnosis

The new classification of neurosis is primarily one of symptoms.
Individually panic, generalized anxiety, hypochondriasis, depressive, phobic and somatoform symptoms can be identified reasonably clearly and have face validity, but they should not be present
too often simultaneously if the classification is to be a useful one.
However, as is well known to every clinician, the simultaneous
presence, or the more ponderous terms, co-occurrence or co-
morbidity, of these symptoms is the rule rather than the exception
(Boyd et al., 1984; Barlow, 1987). Because of this a set of complicated
manoeuvres has to be put into operation to select one of the
symptoms as paramount and the others as secondary ones. In DSM-
III a strict hierarchy was employed in which the place of every
diagnosis was strictly limited in relationship to others above it in the
hierarchy. Thus a patient with classical symptoms of panic disorder

Table 8.2   Hierarchy of neurotic disorders in DSM-III*

| Diagnosis |
| --- |
| Major Depressive Episodes |
| Obsessive–Compulsive Disorder |
| Agoraphobia with Panic Disorder |
| Panic Disorder |
| Agoraphobia Alone, Social Phobia, Simple Phobia |
| Dysthymic Disorder, Somatoform Disorders |
| Generalized Anxiety Disorder |
| Adjustment and Stress Disorders |

* Disorders at the top of this list take precedence over lower ones. In DSM-III-R c
morbidity is allowed.

had to receive a diagnosis of major depressive episode, no matte
how strongly the clinician or investigator felt about the primacy c
panic, if the criteria for major depressive episode were present at th
same time as the panic (Tyrer, 1984a).

Similarly, a patient with long-standing symptoms of generalize
anxiety would have had the diagnosis of generalized anxiety di
order replaced by one of panic disorder if only three panic attack
had just been experienced in the last three weeks. This approach ha
the benefit of simplicity but can only be accepted if it can be show
that the hierarchy is a true one, in which case all patients wit
symptoms at a higher level in the hierarchy should have th
symptoms at lower levels also. This is not always the case and ther
is evidence from both clinical and family studies that patients wit
major depressive episodes, for example, who have symptoms suc
as generalized anxiety and panic also are more handicapped an
have a greater family loading of depressive and anxiety diagnose
than those who have major depressive episodes alone (Weissman
al., 1984). This has been appreciated by the Task Force involved i
revising DSM-III and the hierarchy adopted now is not nearly s
strict as in DSM-III (Table 8.2). If the hierarchy is suspended then th
clinician is faced with a cumbersome list of diagnoses that can b
very confusing. It is natural for some kind of ordering to be invoke
in describing these; the most common is to allow the clinician t
decide whether one disorder is 'due to' another one so that
hierarchy of cause rather than symptomatology is made.

Hierarchies are not necessarily artificial and some system o
diagnostic precedence is often essential and makes good clinica
sense. Thus, for example, it is reasonable for a patient with schizo

phrenia who is anxious about his delusions to have his anxiety relegated by the clinician to a role that is diagnostically insignificant. To a lesser extent the hierarchy of neurotic disorder is understandable. Depression and anxiety are both disorders of mood but even minor degrees of depression cause more problems in social functioning than anxiety (Casey *et al.*, 1985; Fredman *et al.*, 1988; Cassano *et al.*, 1989).

When one diagnosis is always associated with another it is also reasonable to employ a hierarchy. For example, pernicious anaemia and subacute combined degeneration of the spinal cord are clinically different syndromes but as they both result from vitamin $B_{12}$ deficiency they belong to the same diagnosis. There is nothing approaching this degree of certainty with any of the individual neurotic disorders (with only obsessive–compulsive disorders coming close) and so the clinician is left with an unsatisfactory list of names which can be singularly unhelpful. The example of Mrs Green given in the prologue of this book illustrates this problem well.

In DSM-III-R the hierarchy is suspended but is still implicitly present in making a diagnosis with many conditions (e.g. with adjustment disorders, dysthymic disorder and major depressive episode).

The other consistent feature in reviewing the literature is the greater frequency of 'co-morbidity' with more serious disorders. Thus patients with generalized anxiety disorder and simple phobia rarely have additional neurotic diagnoses but those with panic and major depressive episode often have several other conditions.

This supports strongly the position of Foulds (1976) who argued persuasively the case for a hierarchy of personal illness, in which the different levels of the hierarchy were determined by the amount of distress and handicap produced by the disorder, and states of disintegration (e.g. schizophrenia, delusional depression) were placed at the top of the hierarchy and mild diffuse depression and anxiety at the base. Foulds argued that all conditions at higher levels of the hierarchy also included disorders below this level. His view has been supported by several workers using independent approaches. Thus, for example, Prusoff and Klerman (1974) found that although less severe depression and anxiety could be differentiated, it was only because the depressed patients had more symptoms than did the anxious ones; the diagnostic differences were additive rather than qualitative. Once more severe depressive symptoms develop they are placed in a higher tier of the Foulds hierarchy and thus take precedence over any co-existing anxiety symptoms. Although the work of Foulds and his main collaborator, Bedford, has

Table 8.3   Summary of the main differences found between anxiety and depressive disorders by the Newcastle group*

| Symptom | Percentage Incidence | |
| --- | --- | --- |
| | Anxiety | Depression |
| Depression – worse in morning | 11 | 48 |
| – reactive to change | 74 | 41 |
| – early waking | 15 | 55 |
| – suicide: acts | 70 | 37 |
| – retardation | 5 | 48 |
| – delusions | 5 | 17 |
| – panic attacks | 86 | 17 |
| Increased autonomic responses | 74 | 23 |
| Emotional lability | 86 | 52 |
| Dizzy attacks | 68 | 40 |
| Marked agoraphobia | 51 | 2 |
| Marked depersonalization | 36 | 4 |
| Perceptual distortion | 42 | 8 |

* Only items showing significant differences are shown.
(Adapted from Roth *et al.*, 1972.)

produced good data in support of this position these are based on a questionnaire, the Delusions–Symptoms–States Inventory (DSSI) (Bedford *et al.*, 1977), which has not commanded widespread use. Nevertheless, results from many sources have generally supported his position. For example, Tyrer *et al.* (1987) found that phobic patients studied over a two-year-period had more phobic symptoms than depressed and anxious patients but did not differ in respect of anxiety and depressive symptoms. Similar findings to those of Prusoff and Klerman (1974) were obtained when the depressed patients were compared with the anxious ones.

Nevertheless, this overlapping view has its dissenters, the more notable of which are Martin Roth and his colleagues in Newcastle. The conclusions of the 'Newcastle group', as they have been called in the United Kingdom for some time, were that depressive and anxiety syndromes overlapped but were none the less distinctive diagnostic syndromes (Roth *et al.*, 1982). The major work of the Newcastle group was published in a series of papers in 1972 and these are worth examining in detail as they have had a major influence on attitudes to the classification of anxiety and depression. The group examined a consecutive series of 169 patients admitted with anxiety and depressive disorders in the Newcastle area. Using the statistical technique of discriminant functional analysis, they looked at the main clinical features, including symptoms, historical data (e.g. presence or absence of neurotic traits in childhood) and a miscellaneous group of attributes, of which personality status is perhaps the most significant.

The results, illustrated in Table 8.3, demonstrated clear-cut qualitative differences between anxiety and depressive diagnoses. Patients with depressive disorders commonly showed a marked diurnal mood swing, early morning waking and psychomotor retardation and had a higher incidence of delusions than those with anxiety states. Conversely, patients with anxiety states commonly had panic attacks, increased emotional lability, agoraphobia, depersonalization and perceptual disturbances, and a history of dependent personality attributes and neurotic traits in childhood (Roth *et al.*, 1972).

Subsequent work established a clear demarcation between four major diagnoses: depressive psychosis, depressive neurosis, phobias (mainly agoraphobia) and anxiety states (Kerr *et al.*, 1972). By using differential weightings for the different symptoms this distinction was emphasised. Some support for the distinction came from another study by the group in which patients were followed up over a four-year period. Patients with depressive illness showed much greater improvement than those with anxiety states (Schapira *et al.*, 1972). This series of studies represents the peak of differentiation between anxiety and depressive disorders; no one reading them can fail to be impressed by the firmness of the distinctions between the disorders.

Since the introduction of DSM-III there have been many reports comparing symptomatology in the main anxious and depressive subgroups. To some extent these enquiries are tautological: as panic attacks define panic disorder one would not expect to find a high incidence of attacks, for example, in generalized anxiety disorder. Nevertheless, they do have some interest and in many ways reveal common findings (Boyd *et al.*, 1984; Barlow *et al.*, 1986; Breier *et al.*, 1986). As mentioned earlier, these to some extent support Foulds' model in which undifferentiated anxiety and depression constitute the lowest tier and above them are 'formed' symptoms such as phobias, panic attacks and avoidant behaviour (although as Foulds' work pre-dated DSM-III the symptom fit is by no means exact). According to this model all those with symptoms at a higher level have symptoms at a lower level also. This model not only accepts, but embraces, overlap and merely states that those with more serious disorders have extra symptomatology.

These findings are at variance with those of the Newcastle group, even allowing for the transatlantic diagnostic differences, and it is difficult to know why. What was unusual about the patients seen in the Newcastle studies was that they were all inpatients and that anxious patients comprised a significant percentage of them. Uncomplicated anxiety states, however defined, are rarely admitted to hospital (Tyrer, 1982). In general practice, however, anxiety disorders are the most common psychiatric conditions (Dunn, 1983). There are therefore likely to be some important differences between the inpatient population of anxious patients and those with depression. There is also the possibility, although it can be only speculative, that the doctors recording the symptoms in the Newcastle patients were already 'trained' to recognise the differences between anxiety and depressive disorders, and thus identify the characteristic features of each. One of the advantages of structured interviews using the formal operational criteria of DSM-III is that all questions are asked in a systematic way and there is less opportunity for a 'halo' effect to develop. Thus, even though many American investigators are firmly committed to the distinctions made in the DSM-III, their findings show a greater area of overlap than do those of the Newcastle group (e.g. DiNardo *et al.*, 1983; Breier *et al.*, 1985). The criticisms of the hierarchy of DSM-III have been convincing enough for DSM-III-R to allow multiple diagnosis to be made. Quite apart from the overlap between these disorders, the family studies showing a much higher prevalence of similar disorders in family members when several disorders coexist, together with the finding that the other family members have a similar range of disorders (Leckman *et al.*, 1983a, b; Noyes *et al.*, 1986b) have undermined the hierarchy from a different standpoint.

When all the family studies are taken together the findings are consistent and persuasive. The risk of disorder in relatives increases with co-morbidity, at least as far as depression is concerned (Table 8.4). There is some tendency for single disorders to be associated with a higher frequency of the same disorder in relatives but this is small compared with the additive risk of disorder when two DSM-III conditions are present together. Of course the table only deals with one or two co-occurring DSM-III diagnoses. When three or more are present together it is reasonable to expect the incidence of similar disorders in families to be considerably higher. The data in Table 8.4 alone would have been sufficient reason for abandoning the hierarchy of DSM-III.

Can anxiety therefore be reliably distinguished from depression? As a symptom it obviously can, particularly when it is defined using the DSM-III criteria of panic disorder. As a syndrome, however, separation is achieved by statistical sleight of hand or clever use of operational criteria rather than convincing arguments based on

Table 8.4 Summary of findings for family studies of Depression, Panic, Agoraphobia and Generalized Anxiety Disorder

| Proband Group | Diagnostic Status of Relatives (rates per 100)* | | | | | |
|---|---|---|---|---|---|---|
| | Major Depressive Episode | Phobias | Panic | GAD | Alcohol Abuse |
| Normal | Low | Low | Low | Low | Low |
| Panic Disorder | Moderate | Low | High | Moderate | Moderate |
| Agoraphobia | Low | Moderate | Moderate | Moderate | Moderate |
| GAD | Low | Low | Low | Moderate | Low |
| Major Depressive Episode (pure) | Moderate | Low | Low | Low | Moderate |
| Major Depression a Panic Disorder | High | Low | Low | Moderate | High |
| Major Depression a GAD | High | Low | Low | Moderate | Moderate |
| Major Depression a Agoraphobia | Moderate | Low | Low | Low | Moderate |

GAD, Generalized Anxiety Disorder.

* Low = 0–8%; moderate = 9–16%; high = 16–24%; very high = >25%.

(Data derived from studies by Crowe et al., 1983; Harris et al., 1983; Leckman et al., 1983a; Noyes et al., 1983, 1986.)

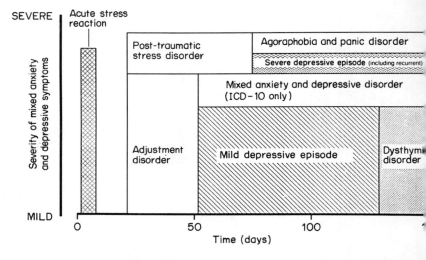

Figure 8.1   The confused classification of mixed anxiety and depressive disorders in DSM–III–R and ICD–10 (the horizontal scale is only approxi mate as many disorders do not have a specified time course)

clinical presentation. The coexistence of anxiety and depressive symptoms is acknowledged by all (even by the Newcastle group in their original studies) but various methods are employed to reduce one at the expense of the other so that either a single diagnosis is made or, if several are necessary, one can be regarded as primary. These techniques have succeeded on the surface as has been illustrated in earlier chapters; mixed anxiety–depressive disorder in ICD-10 and agoraphobia with panic are the only conditions in which mixed pathology is allowed. However, mixed anxiety–depressive disorder is only accepted at a very mild level of pathology and implies that physicians in primary care will encounter it frequently but that practising psychiatrists will not, and, as we have already seen, the similarities between agoraphobia with panic and panic disorder alone are so great that they could almost be merged.

Mixed anxiety–depressive disorder is common (Paykel, 1971) and only a tiny part is reflected in the ICD-10 category. Thus the clinician is warned not to use the diagnosis of mixed anxiety and depressive disorder when symptoms of either type exceed 'mild or moderate degree' and yet to qualify for the diagnosis 'some autonomic symptoms (such as tremor, palpitations, dry mouth, stomach churning etc.) must be present, even if only intermittently; do not use this category if only worry or over-concern are present without auto-nomic symptoms' (World Health Organization, 1988). The clinician is therefore forced to consider patients within a very narrow win-dow of presentation for the diagnosis (Figure 8.1).

A good diagnosis is an economical one. It should be no more than a few words and should describe an exclusive, homogeneous popu-lation. By no stretch of the imagination can panic disorder, major depressive episode, generalised anxiety disorder or dysthymia be regarded as exclusive and homogeneous conditions.

## Stability of diagnosis

We live at a time in which the present dominates past and future in public consciousness almost absolutely. The philosophy of 'short-termism' is a direct consequence; only the immediate future is taken seriously into account in making decisions. For the nosologist this is disturbing. Much greater effort is being put into studying cross-sectional than longitudinal diagnosis and although this has led to an impressive range of published studies their value to the clinician is dubious unless they have the merit of stability.

Such stability need not indicate persistence of an individual diagnosis but any changes should be predictable and linked in an understandable way. Thus the progression of panic disorder to agoraphobia with panic is acceptable provided that panic disorder does indeed have this outcome. The clinician meeting a patient satisfying the diagnostic criteria for panic disorder would then know the likely outcome and its time course in the same way that he could predict the outcome of an untreated patient presenting with a primary syphilitic chancre. The manifestations of the disorder change but this does not negate the diagnosis. Quite apart from changes to another diagnosis the change from a named disorder to resolution (no diagnosis) is obviously a permitted one and is implied in many conditions (e.g. adjustment disorder).

If, however, the patient with panic disorder has one of six possible outcomes of roughly equal representation the diagnosis is of little value to the clinician. The more rapid the transition between diag-nosis the less satisfactory the label becomes. If the change in diagnosis in unpredictable its usefulness is diminished further and there is very little that can be gleaned from the description except present mental state.

The relative stability of each of the main groups of neurotic disorders is summarised in Table 8.5. The most stable diagnosis is one that is persistent, predictable and rarely changes to another

Table 8.5  Stability of major neurotic diagnoses

| Diagnosis | Persistence | Predictability of Diagnostic Outcome | Frequency of Diagnostic Change |
| --- | --- | --- | --- |
| Panic Disorder | Low | Poor | High |
| Generalized Anxiety Disorder | Moderate | Poor | Moderate |
| Agoraphobia with Panic | High | Good | Moderate |
| Agoraphobia without Panic | High | Good | Moderate |
| Social Phobia | High | Good | Low |
| Simple Phobia | Very high | Good | Very low |
| Obsessive–Compulsive Disorder | High | Good | Low |
| Major Depressive Disorder | Low | Good | Moderate |
| Dysthymic Disorder | Moderate | Fair | High |
| Dissociative Disorders | Low | Fair | Moderate |
| Somatoform Disorders | High | Good | Moderate |
| Stress and Adjustment Disorders | Low | Good | Moderate |
| Post-traumatic Stress Disorders | Moderate | Good | Low |

condition. Simple phobia tops the list and panic disorder is at the bottom. Only the phobic and obsessive–compulsive disorders are stable over time but the predictability of the depressive, somatoform and stress disorders improves their diagnostic status to more acceptable levels. The table is based on a series of studies concerned with longitudinal stability (Kendell, 1974; Clancy *et al.*, 1978; Dealy *et al.*, 1981; Munjack and Moss, 1981; Uhde *et al.*, 1985; Breier *et al.*, 1986) together with as yet unpublished data on the stability of panic, dysthymic and generalised anxiety disorders from the Nottingham study of neurotic disorder (Tyrer *et al.*, 1988b).

Unfortunately most of the published work is retrospective which is not surprising in view of the short history of the DSM-III diagnoses. There are many potential distortions in such data, including the tendency we all have to find plausible reasons for change (Frederick Bartlett's (1932) 'effort after meaning'), gender differences in denying and admitting mental health problems (Angst and Dobler-Mikola, 1984) and the diagnostic bias of investigators who may have pre-formed views of diagnostic status. In personal studies we have minimised these by prospective evaluation at frequent intervals by psychiatric assessors who are blind to original diagnostic status.

Many more prospective longitudinal studies are needed to establish whether the findings of Table 8.5 are definitive rather than provisional. Such studies are difficult to mount, are often expensive and their rewards are slow in coming, and so have little to do with 'short-termism'. Nevertheless, they are essential to understanding and will affect diagnostic practice much more than the dozens of cross-sectional sorties into the diagnostic jungle that currently dominate our thinking.

## Time course

Although this is linked to stability it is worth considering separately. As already indicated, the major influence on diagnosis is the nature of the main presenting symptoms. Once a symptom reaches diagnostic status it is used to shuffle conditions into groups. Like the emblems of the four suites in a pack of cards, the major neurotic symptoms, anxiety, depression, obsessions, phobias and somatic complaints, are displayed prominently in every diagnostic member. Dissociative, adjustment and stress disorders are excluded as their symptomatology is more diffuse and diagnosis incorporates the psychosocial stressors involved in precipitating the disorder.

The ground rules for diagnosis therefore seem to be reasonably clear. Unfortunately they are changed frequently, and unsystematically, in making many individual diagnoses. The time course of symptoms necessary to make a diagnosis varies from only a few days in the case of panic disorder (a period of sufficient length to have four panic attacks) to most of the last two years in the case of dysthymic disorder (Table 8.6). If this was applied consistently there would be no problems in diagnosis; we would merely have acute, intermediate and chronic subgroups for all the major symptoms. But it is not applied consistently, and many of the diagnoses appear to have been created speciously in an attempt to achieve separate identity for many conditions which do not deserve such status. In

Table 8.6   Variations in time course between neurotic diagnosis

| Diagnosis | Duration of Symptoms Necessary to Satisfy Diagnosis |
|---|---|
| Acute Stress Reactions (ICD-10 only) | A few hours |
| Adjustment Disorders | Between 0 and 6 months after onset of stressful event |
| Post-traumatic Stress Disorder | 4 weeks |
| Panic Disorder | 4 attacks in any period up to 4 weeks |
| Generalized Anxiety Disorder | 1 month |
| Major Depressive Episode | 2 weeks |
| Dysthymic Disorder | Most of the last 2 years |
| Agoraphobia with and without Panic | Not specified |
| Social and Simple Phobias | Not specified |
| Obsessive–Compulsive Disorder | Not specified (but symptoms have to be recurrent) |
| Dissociative Disorders | Not specified |

short, it looks like cheating. Where are the 'major anxiety episodes' to compare with the major depressive ones; where is generalized (mild) depressive disorder of six to twelve months' duration; and how should acute bouts of depression lasting only a few hours be classified? These questions may appear flippant to those who are so steeped in DSM-III terminology that they have stopped questioning these categories, but they point to the serious omissions in current classification. These undefined conditions appear frequently in clinical practice and can be confirmed by a visit to any psychiatric outpatient clinic. Where symptoms are more distinct and better defined there seems to be no great concern about the duration of symptoms. It is odd that time course has become so important in classifying the anxiety and depressive disorders.

There is another problem introduced by the time factor in the new disorders. If a condition is defined by its duration it is predictable that those diagnoses of short duration will have a better outcome than those that have lasted longer. Whilst this may be justified in the case of adjustment and stress disorders it is unsatisfactory for the others. If dysthymia has a less satisfactory outcome than major depressive episode it can be regarded as a successful diagnosis but the two conditions may only represent the two ends of the same condition. As all mental disorders cover the range between excellent and poor outcome it is a little artificial to incorporate these features into separate diagnoses.

## Treatment response

This is the most important implication of diagnosis for the practising doctor. If the sometimes painful and time-consuming exercise of diagnosis has no treatment implications it may still be important (as for example in the differential diagnosis of dementia) but it ceases to have immediacy in clinical practice and becomes relegated to more academic sidelines. Does the new classification have important treatment implications not possessed by the old?

The recommended treatment for each of the new disorders suggests that the answer to this question is a negative one (Table 8.7). The phobic and obsessional disorders are responsive to various forms of behaviour therapy, notably exposure, that are not appropriate for the others in the group, but for the other diagnoses there is surprising convergence of treatment across all disorders. Pharmacological dissection begins to look like semantic dissection only; although the named disorders look different in their new clothes, underneath they are the same and respond similarly to treatment. From the standpoint of the therapist the treatment of most neurotic disorders could be summarised as 'psychotherapy always, antidepressants sometimes and anti-anxiety drugs sparingly', with little significant modification for each of the different conditions.

Nevertheless, there are some differences in the severity of some diagnoses compared with others. There are many sources of evidence suggesting that panic disorder, for example, is more severe than generalized anxiety disorder. This is shown with regard to its symptoms (Hoehn-Saric, 1982a; Hoehn-Saric and McLeod, 1985) and in perceived need for treatment (Boyd, 1986). If this difference in severity was also associated with differential treatment response the separation of the two diagnoses would be justified.

The evidence does not support such differential response. As already argued, the psychological treatment for panic, generalized anxiety and depression overlap considerably and drug treatments show similar effects. For example, in the Nottingham study of neurotic disorder (Tyrer *et al.*, 1988b) patients with panic disorder, generalized anxiety disorder and dysthymic disorder were treated with cognitive and behaviour therapy, self-help, dothiepin (the most commonly used antidepressant in the United Kingdom),

Table 8.7 Recommended psychological and drug treatments for neurotic disorders

| Diagnosis | Preferred Psychological Treatment | Preferred Pharmacological Treatment |
|---|---|---|
| Acute Stress Reactions | Counselling/support | Benzodiazepines for anxiety (less than one week) Beta-blocking drugs |
| Adjustment Disorders | Counselling and/or psychotherapy | Probably as for acute stress reactions but poor evidence available |
| Agoraphobia | Exposure *in vivo* | Tricyclic antidepressants MAOIs |
| Social Phobia | Exposure *in vivo* Social skills training | Uncertain, but MAOIs and tricyclic antidepressants effective |
| Simple Phobia | Exposure *in vivo* Desensitisation | Not appropriate |
| Generalized Anxiety Disorder | Anxiety management training | Benzodiazepines (acute phase) Tricyclic antidepressants |
| Panic Disorder | Anxiety management training Cognitive therapy | Benzodiazepines (acute phase) Tricyclic antidepressants and MAOIs (chronic) |
| Obsessive–Compulsive Disorder | Exposure *in vivo* | Tricyclic antidepressants |
| Major Depressive Episode | Cognitive therapy | Tricyclic antidepressants |

MAOI, monoamine oxidase inhibitor

diazepam or placebo over a six-week period and this was then reduced and withdrawn by ten weeks. The results showed that diazepam was significantly worse than the other treatments and that those allocated to placebo had significantly more additional treatment during the ten-week period. However, diagnosis had no significant influence on response. The only significant finding was that generalised anxiety disorder was less severe than panic disorder in terms of anxiety symptoms and that dysthymic disorder

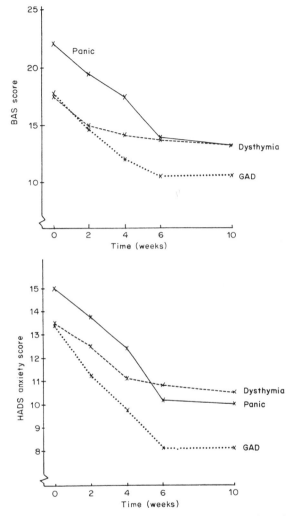

Figure 8.2   Anxiety symptoms in patients with panic disorder ($n = 73$), generalized anxiety disorder (GAD) ($n = 65$) and dysthymic disorder ($n = 63$) after ten weeks of drug or psychological treatment. Symptoms measured by the Brief Scale for Anxiety (BAS) (Tyrer *et al.*, 1984) and by the anxiety part of the Hospital Anxiety and Depression Scale (HADS) (Zigmond and Snaith, 1983). Patients with panic disorder and dysthymic disorder have significantly higher scores than those with GAD ($p = 0.015$). (From Tyrer *et al.*, 1988b. Reproduced by permission of the Editor and Publishers of the *Lancet*)

responded less well than the other two diagnoses (Figure 8.2). As the degree of improvement was the most similar between panic and generalized anxiety disorder and as the requirements for the diagnosis of dysthymic disorder tended to pre-select a poor-responding group (p. 144) there is little in these results to support separate diagnosis of the three groups.

The sad conclusion to be drawn from these enquiries is that the new diagnostic systems have been of no benefit to the clinician. This conclusion hardly seems credible in view of the tremendous research interests that have been generated by the classifications, but the therapeutic advances implied by the diagnostic reformulation have not materialised.

This would not assume such prominence if treatment had not already been highlighted as an important reason for reclassifying the neurotic disorders. As indicated in earlier chapters the main stimulus behind the introduction of panic disorder as a separate diagnosis was the suggestion that it was a syndrome specifically responsive to antidepressants (Klein, 1981). This has now been shown to be wrong, yet panic disorder has developed a momentum of its own and will not be stopped easily.

One of the strongest reasons for separating anxiety and depressive disorders was the difference in treatment implied by the two conditions. A generation of psychiatrists and doctors in training have been taught to recognise the clinical distinctions between the two disorders because of their alleged importance in treatment. Apart from separating milder forms of depression from delusional depression and other forms with marked biological features the exercise has proved of little therapeutic value. In particular, the common 'neurotic' forms of depression show no therapeutic distinction from the 'neurotic' forms of anxiety. Almost invariably there are admixtures of both groups of symptoms in all patients and the allocation of diagnosis is almost a random exercise. What has tended to happen over the last 25 years is that diagnosis has been made to justify a chosen treatment rather than treatment following naturally from the diagnosis. With the introduction of antidepressants to clinical practice many conditions formerly diagnosed as anxiety states were now diagnosed as depressive disorders in order to justify treatment with the new drugs.

The absence of therapeutic distinction between anxiety and depressive disorders indicates that reluctance to diagnose a mixed anxiety–depressive group of disorders is no longer valid. The additional evidence that 'anxious depressions' have a worse outcome than other depressive disorders also supports the case for a mixed syndrome.

## Personality status

One of the most important consequences of the introduction of DSM-III was the description of mental disorders under five axes, of which the first two are the mental state and personality status. This emphasised an issue in classification that was in danger of being forgotten. Individuals can have one of four possible diagnostic states: no mental state or personal disorder, mental state disorder with normal personality, personality disorder with normal mental state, and simultaneous mental state and personality disorder. This was in danger of being overlooked because of the clinical tendency to diagnose patients as having either a mental state abnormality *or* a personality disorder.

One of the negative aspects of this separation is that there is no provision for combining disorders of mental state and personality, the important fourth group in the above list. This is understandable but is misleading if certain types of personality abnormality are *consistently* associated with particular disorders of mental state.

In the case of the neurotic disorders there is a large body of evidence providing consistent findings over many years concerning the association of neurotic symptomatology with a certain type (or types) of abnormal personality.

This was well described in the early psychoanalytical literature and perhaps encapsulated in Franz Alexander's (1930) description of the 'neurotic character'. Subsequently both psychodynamic and biologically orientated psychiatrists have found that dependent, inhibited and anxious personalities, also described as oral personalities, are very common in patients diagnosed as having a neurotic disorder (Horney, 1939; Fromm, 1942; Slater, 1943; Paykel *et al.*, 1973; Lazare *et al.*, 1976; Mann *et al.*, 1981b; Friedman *et al.*, 1985; Tyrer *et al.*, 1986). These studies have also demonstrated that antisocial and schizoid personality features are less marked than the other psychiatric populations. There is some evidence that these personality characteristics are more marked in the anxiety disorders and that obsessional personality features are more prominent in obsessive–compulsive disorder (Tyrer *et al.*, 1983), but in general the common features are far more prominent than their differences.

Not only are dependent and inhibited personalities more likely to be associated with neurotic disorder than other types of abnormal personality, but there is a high rate of co-occurrence of personality abnormality and mental state. Nearly 40% of psychiatric outpatients with neurotic disorders have significant personality disturbance (Tyrer *et al.*, 1983), although the proportion falls to between 15%

and 30% in patients with neurotic disorders in primary care (Mann *et al.*, 1981a; Casey *et al.*, 1984; Casey, 1986). These percentages may surprise some readers. Early studies generally found low rates of personality disorder in primary care, outpatient and hospital populations: rarely higher than 10% (Cooper, 1965; Shepherd *et al.*, 1966; Muller et al., 1967). However, these studies were carried out at a time when personality disorder was considered to be an *alternative* to, rather than associated with, mental state disorders and predated formal assessment of personality status (Casey and Tyrer, 1986; Casey, 1988).

In general, studies have found greater personality abnormality in phobic, obsessional and anxiety disorders than in depressive ones (Roth *et al.*, 1972, 1982; Tyrer *et al.*, 1983; Casey *et al.*, 1984). Dependent personality traits are amongst the criteria suggested by the Newcastle group for separating anxiety and depression. However, it has already been noted in previous chapters that there is some difficulty in separating dependent personality features from anxious symptoms, and avoidant personality features from phobic ones, and even with structured interview schedules it is not possible to remove this overlap entirely. The overall association of personalilty disorder with neurotic disturbance is remarkably similar between the different neurotic diagnoses (Tyrer *et al.*, 1988a, pp. 102–3). For those with personality disturbance the term 'chronic neurosis' is often applied, and this is exemplified by the case of Mrs Green described in the prologue of this book.

Any clinician or researcher studying neurotic disorders cannot ignore associated personality disturbance. A case can therefore be made for including this in classification and making a distinction between those patients with neurotic conditions who have no personality disturbance and those who do.

## INTEGRATION OF ANXIETY AND DEPRESSIVE SYMPTOMS

There are many reasons for trying to separate anxiety from depression. They are different mood states with qualitatively distinct biological functions; they involve different neurotransmitters (Hoehn-Saric, 1982; Heninger and Charney, 1987) and have different antecedents. Depression tends to follow loss and 'exit' events (Paykel *et al.*, 1969), whilst anxiety is a response to uncertainty and to danger (Finlay-Jones and Brown, 1981). What, therefore, is the point of trying to bring them together in a single condition? Is it, as Klein and Klein (1989a) assert, just an example of 'perfectionistic paralysis', the refusal to make these states distinct only because their 'level of fit' as separate conditions is not quite right? The plaudits are reserved for those who make a success of the distinction because this seems to be the correct form of classification. Conversely, evidence that fails to show a distinction is looked on with suspicion as unsound and inadequate in some way, sometimes even regarded as unscientific as well as unhelpful.

These are prejudices that do not help understanding. How things are are seldom what they should be to the pigeon-holer. The important issue is not whether it is possible to draw a line of distinction between anxiety and depression but whether this distinction is useful in clinical practice (Kendell, 1975). A line can be drawn, albeit a somewhat wobbly, convoluted one, between these conditions (Roth *et al.*, 1972; Roth and Mountjoy, 1982) but the conditions so separated do not retain their distinction for long. The situation is analogous to a snapshot of a pair of identical twins. By close examination it is possible to identify some distinguishing characteristics, a small difference in weight, hair length or posture, and if one or more of these is given special significance they may continue to maintain their distinction for some time later. But most observers will fail to make the distinction and continue to regard the two as identical. Twins, like anxiety and depression, are under constant pressures to diverge from their natural similarity and, as a consequence, many do so to some extent, but revert later when the pressures have been removed. (I write from experience as a monozygotic twin.) Anxiety and depressive disorders are similar: they can be distinguished by expert observers, but for most purposes are too similar to be separated as distinct diagnostic groups.

As anxiety and depression are so highly correlated it could be argued that all disorders in which these symptoms are prominent are mixed ones and should be classified accordingly. At the extreme ends of the spectrum of these disorders, however, there are important changes, mainly in behaviour, that affect presentation and classification. Severe depressive illness is associated with the biological concomitants of weight and appetite loss and psychomotor retardation, which are physiologically opposed to the changes of anxiety (Noble and Lader, 1972). At the other extreme, severe anxiety leads to avoidance and thence to phobias. Once phobias are established they tend to persist and dominate the clinical picture, as do obsessional symptoms once established fully. This is acknowledged by Foulds (1979) in his hierarchical model, in which phobias and obsessions take precedence over diffuse anxiety and depressive symptoms, and by Marks (1987) in his classificatory group of 'anxious avoidant' disorders, which includes both obsessional and

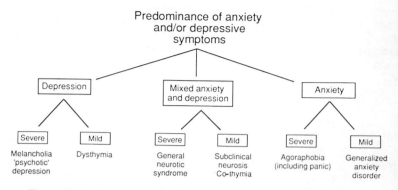

Figure 8.3   A suggested classification of anxiety and depression

phobic disorders. At the mild end of the anxiety spectrum we have the adjustment and stress disorders. It is interesting that classifications have long been happy to include mixed affective symptoms in these groups, including panic as well as anxiety and depression, without the diagnosis being contradicted. Although, as discussed earlier in this chapter, there are some handicaps to setting time limits to these diagnoses in advance the great importance of psychosocial stresses in inducing mixed neurotic symptoms deserves mention and is justified in these diagnoses.

In the neurotic disorders mixed symptoms are the norm. Whilst this is disturbing for the classifier it is worse to pretend that overlap is insignificant and to separate these mood states in a contrived manner. It was attempted in DSM-III and failed. If one accepts that the mixed anxiety and depression mule is neither an anxious horse nor a depressive donkey and, like anxiety and depression, can be separated into mild and severe groups, six conditions are delineated (Figure 8.3). Obvious synonyms for the severe and mild depressive disorders are listed in Figure 8.3 and reflect the long-standing argument over the classification of depression. In the latest classifications this division is best represented by the ICD-10 categories; DSM-III-R appears unduly convoluted and confused with no clear level of demarcation and the continuation of the unsatisfactory criteria for major depressive disorder allow a larger number of individuals whom the average clinical psychiatrist would not regard as markedly depressed to be included in this category. For those with predominant anxiety there is a distinction between the more severe forms that demonstrate the symptom of panic and, almost invariably, symptoms of phobic avoidance and fear. Panic is not included as a separate category because of its extremely close connections with agoraphobia. Mild anxiety is equivalent to the category of generalised anxiety disorder in both current classifications.

Mixed anxiety and depression is already recognised in its mild form in ICD-10 and is described as common in the population at large and in primary-care settings. This is similar to the 'sub-clinical neurosis' of Taylor and Chave (1964) in their pioneering epidemiological survey of mental health in a new town. An alternative synonym is 'co-thymia', so named because it indicates the coming together of two moods in a single diagnosis. The more severe form of mixed anxiety and depression is, for reasons discussed below, described as the general neurotic syndrome.

The groups outlined in Figure 8.3 are diagnostic hypotheses that need testing in practice. For reasons already given, there is some doubt about the validity of mild depressive and anxiety diagnoses because of the almost invariable overlap between anxiety and depression at less severe levels of pathology. Nevertheless, they deserve to be considered equally until tested fully and it is quite possible that separate disorders in these categories can be identified even after acknowledging the existence of a co-thymia group. It is worth reminding the reader that all the diagnoses in ICD-10 and DSM-III-R are working hypotheses, and invite the investigator to test their validity from the standpoints of aetiology, stability, response to treatment and long-term development. However, such has been the short-term success of introducing clearer diagnostic criteria that every diagnosis gets the stamp of validity by merely being included in the lists. Some are confirmed in their diagnostic position while others are rejected as a consequence of enquiry; the same should apply to the mixed anxiety–depressive disorders.

## IDENTIFICATION OF THE GENERAL NEUROTIC SYNDROME

It should not be assumed that permission to grant mixed anxiety–depressive disorders diagnostic status will sabotage the current classification of neurotic disorders and deny alternatives. The general neurotic syndrome is a diagnosis that has both inclusion and exclusion criteria and is not made lightly. The aim of the diagnosis is to identify the core of neurosis exemplified by all the features implied by the term in the prologue of this book.

The procedure for classifying the syndrome involves the demonstration of primary anxiety and depressive symptoms that show changes in primacy at different times, are manifest in the absence of major life events and which commonly occur against a background of personality disturbance in which dependent and/or inhibited qualities are prominent. It is also likely that there will be a positive family history of a similar condition.

## Procedure for the diagnosis of the general neurotic syndrome

The general neurotic syndrome is characterised by the simultaneous presence of various anxiety and depressive symptoms occurring in the absence of major psychological or physical trauma in individuals who have inhibited or dependent personalities. The diagnosis is made through a three-stage process:

(1) identification of the co-occurrence of anxiety and depressive symptoms in the absence of severe depressive illness and other significant psychiatric disorder;
(2) examination of environmental precipitants of these symptoms and measurement of their severity;
(3) determination of the premorbid personality of the subject.

### Co-occurrence of Anxiety and Depressive Symptoms

The patient has evidence of pathological anxiety and depression with a minimum duration of four weeks and manifest by the following:

(1) anxiety demonstrated in the form of the following: (i) acute attacks of panic occurring together with fear of personal catastrophe and/or (ii) persistent anxiety and tension sufficient to cause distress and impaired social and occupational performance. Bodily symptoms commonly occur with this degree of anxiety and include: (i) muscular tension, (ii) headache, (iii) tremor, (iv) chest, neck or other muscular pains, (v) racing of the heart, (vi) palpitations, (vii) sweating, (viii) nausea, (ix) abdominal churning or discomfort, (x) difficulty in breathing, (xi) choking sensations, (xii) dizziness or faintness, (xiii) urinary frequency. The number of symptoms possessed is not critical but the clinician has to be satisfied that they are serious enough to cause impaired performance as described above.

(2)   depressive symptoms of lowered mood, feelings of pessimism about the future, lack of energy, suicidal thoughts and morbid preoccupation (but not associated with significant weight loss (greater than 10 kg), psychomotor retardation, early morning waking, diurnal mood swing or delusions, hallucinations and severe agitation).

Both anxiety and depressive symptoms should normally have been present for at least part of the day, on every day, during the past four weeks.

## Change in Primacy of Depressive and Anxiety Symptoms

Examination of the past history reveals differences in the severity of depressive and anxiety symptoms at different times with at least one occasion in which the primacy of these symptoms is reversed from that at present (e.g. if depressive symptoms are currently the most dominant feature there have been times in the past when anxiety or panic have predominated). The changes in primacy should also have lasted for a minimum of four weeks.

## Absence of Major Psychological or Physical Trauma

If all the symptoms noted above are immediately related in time to major trauma and have not occurred previously, except in response to trauma of equivalent severity, the diagnosis is more likely to be that of an adjustment reaction and not general neurotic syndrome. If the onset of symptoms is within four weeks of a major personally significant event and no previous symptoms have occurred, the criteria for a diagnosis of general neurotic syndrome have not been met. Personally significant events can include major loss (including work, close relative, prized possession, close friend or pet) and major threat (serious or suspected major physical illness, personal danger or threat to personal status and lifestyle, e.g. financial collapse). However, the exact nature of the event and threat must be taken in the context of the subject's value system in judging its severity.

   If the symptoms have persisted for longer than six months after a major traumatic event has ceased the diagnosis of general neurotic syndrome can be made provided the other criteria for diagnosis are satisfied.

## Absence of Persistent Avoidant or Compulsive Behaviour

The mixed anxiety and depressive symptoms are not associated with persistent avoidant or compulsive behaviour. Coexistence of phobic anxiety (sitiuationally predisposed fear) and obsessive–compulsive symptoms (thought, ideas or behaviour) normally invalidates the diagnosis of general neurotic syndrome unless such symptoms (1) last for four weeks or less or (2) are not associated with continuous avoidance of certain situations (apart from well-circumscribed ones such as animals, height, thunder etc. that allow an additional diagnosis of simple phobia to be made).

## Personality Status

The aim is to make an independent assessment of personality that is in no way contaminated by present symptomatology. In some cases this can be achieved with the subject but, wherever possible, information should be derived from an informant who knows the patient well. To satisfy the criteria for the general neurotic syndrome subjects must show evidence of inhibited or dependent personality traits as primary personality features. These are summarised below:

(1)  inhibited traits: the presence of rigidity, preoccupations with detail, restricted emotional expression with self-consciousness and low self-esteem;
(2)  dependent traits: lacking in resources, inability or reluctance to make decisions without other's help, submissiveness and childishness.

These features have to be present in sufficient degree to lead to impairment of social functioning to such a level that they can at least be regarded as constituting personality difficulty, if not personality disorder.

These characteristics are included under dependent and obsessive–compulsive (anankastic) personality disorders in ICD-10 and DSM-III-R and are summarised in Table 8.8.

The diagnostic procedure may be enhanced by using structured interviews for mental state disorders such as the Schedule for Affective Disorders and Schizophrenia (Spitzer and Endicott, 1983), the Present State Examination (Wing *et al.*, 1974), the Structured Clinical Interview for DSM-III-R (Spitzer *et al.*, 1987), or the Composite International Diagnostic Interview (Robins *et al.*, 1988) although the timescales indicated for some diagnoses (e.g. major depressive episode) will need adjusting to the four-week interval

Table 8.8  Classification of inhibited and dependent personality characteristics in DSM-III-R and ICD-10

| Group | DSM-III-R | ICD-10 |
|---|---|---|
| Inhibited | Obsessive–compulsive: pervasive perfectionism, inflexibility, rigidity | Anankastic: indecisiveness, doubt, excessive caution, pedantry, rigidity, need to plan in excessive detail |
| | Avoidant: pervasive social discomfort, fear of negative evaluation, timidity | Anxious: persistent tension, self-consciousness, exaggeration of risks and dangers, restricted lifestyle, hypersensitivity to rejection |
| Dependent | Dependent: persistent dependent and submissive behaviour | Dependent: failure to take responsibility for actions, subordination of personal needs to those of others, excessive dependence, need for constant reassurance, feelings of helplessness whenever a close relationship ends |

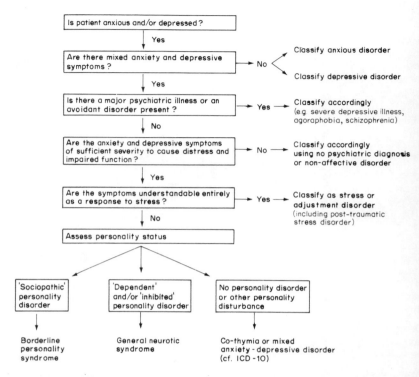

Figure 8.4   Flow chart for classifying anxiety and depressive symptoms

given above and the hierarchy giving precedence of depression over anxiety in many instruments has to be suspended. Diagnosis may also be assisted by formal assessment of personality status using instruments such as the Personality Assessment Schedule (Tyrer and Alexander, 1979; Tyrer *et al.*, 1988); the Standardized Assessment of Personality (Mann *et al.*, 1981b), which has been recently updated to include DSM-III-R and ICD-10 diagnoses; the Structured Interview for the DSM-III Personality Disorders (Pfohl *et al.*, 1982; Stangl *et al.*, 1985); or the Personality Disorder Examination (Loranger *et al.*, 1985), which has also been updated to record both ICD and DSM revisions. For the purposes of diagnosis of the general neurotic syndrome the lesser degree of personality abnormality, personality difficulty (Tyrer *et al.*, 1988) can also be recorded and if dependent or anankastic features are primary the diagnosis of

Table 8.9   A scale for the diagnosis of the general neurotic syndrome

| Positive Features | Score | Negative Features | Score |
|---|---|---|---|
| Simultaneous presence of anxiety and depressive symptoms, each sufficiently severe to qualify for a formal anxiety and depressive diagnosis* and normally lasting for two months or longer | +2 | Persistent phobic or obsessional symptoms for three months or longer | −2 |
| At least one change in primacy of anxiety and depressive symptoms at different times in the course of the disorder | +3 | Anxiety and depressive symptoms only presenting within one month of major life stresses or events | −3 |
| Co-occurrence of phobic, panic, obsessional or hypochondriacal symptoms of variable severity, but not persisting for longer than three months | +1 | | |
| Dependent or anxious (avoidant) premorbid personality disorder* | +3 | Antisocial, histrionic, impulsive or borderline personality disorder* | −3 |
| Anankastic (obsessive–compulsive) personality disorder* | +1 | | |
| At least one first-degree relative has a similar mixed anxiety-depressive disorder | +2 | | |

* Using ICD-10 or DSM-III-R criteria.
Total score of 6 or more: definite syndrome.
Total score of 4–5: possible syndrome.

general neurotic syndrome can be supported.

There have been valid criticisms of the current classificatory system of personality disorder (Rutter, 1987) and the problem of multiple diagnoses has not been resolved adequately. In severe personality disorders, as for example in a forensic population (Mbatia and Tyrer, 1988), it is common to find patients satisfying the criteria for four or more different personality disorders and unless there is a system for grading the degree of severity (as for example in the Personality Assessment Schedule and the Standardized Assessment of Personality) it is difficult to decide which is primary. This is important for classification of mixed anxiety–depressive disorders for sociopathic personality characteristics, included in ICD-10 and DSM-III-R under the headings of dyssocial (antisocial), impulsive borderline, and, to a lesser degree, histrionic and narcissistic personality disorder, are not part of the general neurotic syndrome they belong to a different group and the title of borderline syndrome may be appropriate for it (Figure 8.4). The main features of this group include the personality characteristics of borderline disorder together with mixed affective symptoms, particularly depression, that are an essential part of the diagnosis and incorporated into its operational criteria (American Psychiatric Association, 1987).

The full procedure for classifying mixed anxiety–depressive disorders is outlined in Figure 8.4. It represents a new departure in diagnosis as it is a co-axial system involving both mental state and personality features. It acknowledges that mixed anxiety and depressive *symptoms* are extremely common and that one needs other information before a satisfactory diagnosis can be made. An alternative approach is to use a scale in which each of the important aspects of the general syndrome is given an appropriate weight (Table 8.9). This allows a simple classification of definite, possible or no general neurotic syndrome.

## GENETIC ASPECTS OF MIXED ANXIETY–DEPRESSIVE DISORDERS

In Chapter 3 the genetic studies of Torgersen (1983) and others were discussed in relationship to panic disorder in particular. These at first sight suggest that panic disorder is inherited specifically and therefore promote its status as a separate diagnosis.

However, there are other data, and other interpretations of Torgersen's findings, that conflict strongly with his conclusions that panic, and not generalized anxiety disorder, is genetically transmitted. The strong evidence of hereditability for the original diagnosis of 'anxiety neurosis' (Slater and Shields, 1969; Noyes *et al.*, 1978) and anxiety symptoms in general (Young *et al.*, 1971) is unlikely to be explained solely by the proportion of patients with panic disorder subsumed within this group. The genetic factors determining the inheritance of panic are probably the same as those responsible for the inheritance of neuroticism, and are not specific to panic (Jardine *et al.*, 1984; Martin *et al.*, 1988). If panic disorder was genetically determined but other anxiety disorders were not, twin studies

Table 8.10 Psychiatric diagnoses of 61 proband twins with anxiety disorders and the diagnosis of their co-twins

| Diagnosis of proband | Diagnosis of Co-twin | | | |
|---|---|---|---|---|
| | Panic | Anxiety (minus panic) | Other Mental Disorders | None |
| Panic (MZ twin) | 4 | 2 | 1 | 6 |
| GAD (MZ twin) | 0 | 2 | 3 | 7 |
| Panic (DZ twin) | 0 | 4 | 1 | 11 |
| GAD (DZ twin) | 2 | 2 | 5 | 11 |

GAD, Generalized Anxiety Disorder; MZ monozygotic; DZ, dizygotic.
(From Torgersen, 1983.)

would show MZ–DZ differences for panic disorder but not for other anxiety diagnoses.

When all the data are examined the evidence of specific genetic contributions to named DSM-III and DSM-III-R disorders is slight. There is overlap between disorders in the neurotic spectrum (including obsessive–compulsive disorder) and disturbing variability in the data from different centres. First-degree relatives should have the same risk of developing disorder as DZ twins, yet the concordance rates for such relatives are up to twice those in the genetic data (Cloninger et al., 1981).

Torgersen's results can easily be interpreted as supporting the notion that anxiety is a hereditable mood with no specific predisposition for any one disorder. His results appear to demonstrate that panic disorder shows genetic effects but that generalized anxiety disorder does not (Table 8.10). However, the key results demonstrating the MZ–DZ differences with panic involve very small numbers and use a definition of panic that was extremely broad. To qualify for inclusion in the panic group each twin only had to have had one panic attack at any time in the past. Quite apart from the potential errors involved in retrospective lifetime diagnosis this very low threshold means that many patients with a DSM-III diagnosis of generalized anxiety disorder could qualify for the panic group using Torgersen's criteria.

A much larger study of 446 twin pairs, as yet unpublished, carried out in Australia shows no evidence that any of the anxiety disorders are inherited specifically. The results support the hypothesis that there is a common diathesis to anxiety that can be manifest as any of the anxiety disorders in the new classification (Andrews, personal communication). This is a crucial issue. Klein and Klein (1988b, p. 175) state 'if Panic Disorder is genetically discrete this cuts through arguments based on clinical observations, history etc., and renders nonsensical claims that spontaneous panic is simply severe anxiety'. Although they then argue that panic is indeed genetically discrete the evidence in favour is flimsy at best and faulty at worst.

The same conclusion follows from examination of data from family studies. When these are taken together (Table 8.4) they show only a small tendency for relatives to have the same disorder as the index cases. What is much more striking is the higher rate of all neurotic disorders in the relatives, and this is increased further when mixed anxiety and depressive disorders are considered. Far from supporting the DSM classification the genetic and family evidence goes a long way towards undermining its specificity and promoting the concept of genetic vulnerability to both anxiety and depressive disorders.

If the genetic data are broadened to include anxiety disorders in general and also the concept of mixed conditions they support a general hereditability model. Those susceptible to anxiety and depressive symptoms through genetic vulnerability are likely to have episodes independently of major life events, to have frequent recurrences and a generally poorer prognosis than other disorders with similar symptoms. The personality features may also be genetically determined.

All these features are part of the concept of the general neurotic syndrome (Tyrer, 1985, 1986a, 1986b, 1989) and for this reason the family history of a similar disorder is supportive of the diagnosis (Table 8.10). The full procedure for making the diagnosis is therefore a composite one involving the identification of symptoms, their precipitants and history, personality assessment and family history.

## 'LUMPERS' VERSUS 'SPLITTERS'

I am well aware that there are natural differences between individuals that affect what can be termed the philosophy of classification. Some are optimistic about its value and are always looking for greater precision by the introduction of new reliable categories. These 'splitters' are offset by the 'lumpers', who tend to be more pessimistic about the value of classification and for whom the common features of different conditions are more important than the criteria that divide them.

This affects the interpretation of data and can lead to an unsatisfactory level of debate in which, no matter the power of the arguments put forward by one side, the other will disagree, and successful persuasion is rare. Thus, a statement such as one by Sir

Martin Roth (1983) that 'systematic investigations of the relationship between anxiety and depressive states . . . have shown the two groups of syndromes to be distinct, with some measure of overlap', is a Delphic statement open to different interpetation. The 'split-ers', of whom Roth is one, can emphasise the points of distinction whereas the 'lumpers' can point to the overlap as being of primary mportance.

This debate tends to become artificial if it becomes removed from clinical practice. Academics can argue for hours about the merits of different systems of classification but unless the clinicians will use hem they have no value. We have to acknowledge that large numbers of clinicians treating neurotic patients are unhappy about heir classification and in many cases abandon the exercise al-ogether. This particularly applies to those who practice psycho-herapy rather than other forms of treatment. Jung's pithy summary of the value of diagnosis in neurotic disorders, although written in 1945, strikes a resonant chord with many clinicians today:

> Diagnosis is a highly irrelevant affair since, apart from affixing a more or less lucky label to a neurotic condition, nothing is gained by it, least of all as regards prognosis and therapy. In flagrant contrast to the rest of medicine, where a definite diagnosis is often, as it were, logically followed by a specific therapy and a more or less certain prognosis, the diagnosis of any particular psychoneurosis means, at most, that some form of psychotherapy is indicated. Nor should we gloss over the fact that the classification of the neuroses is very unsatisfactory and that for this reason alone a specific diagnosis seldom means anything real. I have in the course of years accustomed myself wholly to disregard the diagnosing of specific neuroses, and have sometimes found myself in a quandary when some word-addict urged me to hand him a specific diagnosis. The Greco-Latin compounds needed for this still seem to have a not inconsiderable market value and are occasionally indispensable for that reason. (Jung, 1954, p. 86)

Unfortunately the current classifications of a neurosis, despite their spurious science, have not progressed much since these words were written. The 'market value' of diagnosis is often high, par-ticularly for research workers in the United States, and firm diag-noses continue to impress patients (at least at first), but their long-term clinical value remains dubious.

It is this issue, rather than arguments between 'lumpers' and 'splitters', that should be occupying our attention and which has prompted the diagnostic suggestions made in this chapter. If we can bring all practitioners, from analytic psychotherapists through to psychopharmacologists, to adopt a common classification because it

makes sense to them in their clinical practice, then we can afford t
be satisfied. Changes that involve recognition of the univers
coexistence of anxiety and depression in neurotic disorders, an
their frequent associations with abnormal personality, only reflec
clinical awareness and need to be recognised in any comprehensiv
classification. Whether such classification leads to one, two or te
different diagnoses is unimportant, but they must be stable con
ditions that have a longer timespan in clinical consciousness tha
some of the names that have been generated frenetically in the pas
ten years.

# Bibliography

Ackner B (1959). Depersonalisation 1. Aetiology and phenomenology. 11. Clinical syndromes. *Journal of Mental Science* **100**, 838–72.

Agras WS (1985a). *Panic: Facing Fears, Phobias, and Anxiety*. New York: Freeman.

Agras WS (1985b). Stress, panic, and the cardiovascular system. In: *Anxiety and the Anxiety Disorders* (eds AH Tuma and JD Maser), pp. 363–68. Hillsdale, NJ: Erlbaum.

Agras WS, Chapin HN and Oliveau DC (1972). The natural history of phobia, *Archives of General Psychiatry* **26**, 315–17.

Akiskal HS (1983). Dysthymic disorder: psychopathology of proposed chronic depressive subtypes. *American Journal of Psychiatry*, **140**, 11–20.

Akiskal HS (1987). The boundaries of mood disorders: implications for defining temperamental variants, atypical subtypes, and schizoaffective disorder. In: *Diagnosis and Classification in Psychiatry: A Critical Appraisal of DSM-III* (ed. G Tischler), pp. 61–93. Cambridge: Cambridge University Press.

Akiskal HS (1989). Validating affective personality types. In: *The Validity of Psychiatric Diagnosis* (ed. L Robins) New York: Raven Press.

Akiskal HS, Djenderedjian AH, Rosenthal RH *et al.* (1977). Cyclothymic disorder: validating criteria for inclusion in the bipolar affective group. *American Journal of Psychiatry* **134**, 1227–33.

Akiskal HS, Bitar AH, Puzantian VR, Rosenthal TL and Walker PW (1978). The nosological status of neurotic depression. *Archives of General Psychiatry* **35**, 756–66.

Akiskal HS, Rosenthal TL, Haykal RF, Lemmi H, Rosenthal RH *et al.*, (1980). Characterological depressions: clinical and sleep EEG findings separating 'subaffective dysthymias' from 'character spectrum disorders'. *Archives of General Psychiatry* **37**, 777–83.

Alexander F (1930). The neurotic character. *International Journal of Psycho analysis* **11**, 291–311.

American Psychiatric Association (1980). *Diagnostic and Statistical Manual of Mental Disorders*, 3rd edn. Washington DC: American Psychiatric Association.

American Psychiatric Association (1987). *Diagnostic and Statistical Manual of Mental Disorders*, revised 3rd edn. Washington DC: American Psychiatric Association.

Ananth J, Pecknold J, Van Den Steen N and Engelsmann FC (1981). Double blind comparative study of clomipramine and amitriptyline in obsessive neurosis. *Progress in Neuro-Psychopharmacology* **5**, 257–62.

Anderson DJ, Noyes R Jr and Crowe RR (1984). A comparison of panic disorder and generalized anxiety disorder. *American Journal of Psychiatry* **141**, 572–5.

Angst J, Baastrup P, Grof P, Hippius H et al. (1973). The course of monopolar depression and bipolar psychoses. *Psychiatria, Neurologia, Neurochirurgia (Amsterdam)* **76**, 489–500.

Angst J and Dobler-Mikola (1984). Do the diagnostic criteria determine the sex-ratio in depression? *Journal of Affective Disorders* **7**, 189–98.

Aronson TA and Logue CM (1987). On the longitudinal course of panic disorder: developmental history and predictors of phobic complications. *Comprehensive Psychiatry* **28**, 344–5.

Åsberg M, Montgomery SA, Perris C, Schalling D and Sedvall G (1978). A comprehensive psychopathological rating scale. *Acta Psychiatrica Scandinavica*, Suppl. 271, 5–29.

Ashcroft G et al. (Chairman M Lader) (1987). Consensus statement: panic disorder. *British Journal of Psychiatry*, **150**, 557–8.

Avery D and Winokur G (1977). The efficacy of electroconvulsive therapy and antidepressants in depression. *Biological Psychiatry* **12**, 507–24.

Ballenger JC, Burrows GD, DuPont RL, Lesser IM, Noyes R Jr et al. (1988). Alprazolam in panic disorder and agoraphobia: results from a multicentre trial. I. Efficacy in short-term treatment. *Archives of General Psychiatry* **45** 413–22.

Barlow DH (1985). The dimensions of anxiety disorders. In: *Anxiety and the Anxiety Disorders* (eds AH Tuma and JD Maser), pp. 479–500. Hillsdale NJ: Erlbaum.

Barlow DH (1987). The classification of anxiety. In: *Diagnosis and Classification in Psychiatry: A Critical Appraisal of DSM-III* (ed. G Tischler), pp. 221–42. Cambridge, Cambridge University Press.

Barlow DH (1988). *Anxiety and its Disorders: The Nature and Treatment of Anxiety and Panic*, New York: Guilford Press.

Barlow DH, Cohen AS, Waddell M, Vermilyea JA, Klosko JS et al. (1984). Panic and generalized anxiety disorders: nature and treatment. *Behavior Therapy* **15**, 431–49.

Barlow DH, Di Nardo PA, Vermilyea BB, Vermilyea JA and Blanchard EB (1986). Co-morbidity and depression among the anxiety disorders: issues in diagnosis and classification. *Journal of Nervous and Mental Disease* **174** 63–72.

Barlow DH and Cerny J (1988). *Psychological Treatment of Panic*. New York: Guilford Press.

Barsky AJ and Klerman GL (1983). Overview: hypochondriasis, bodily complaints, and somatic styles. *American Journal of Psychiatry* **140**, 273–83.

Bartlett FC (1932). *Remembering: A Study of Experimental and Social Psychology*. London: Cambridge University Press.

Bayer R and Spitzer RL (1985). Neurosis, psychodynamics and DSM-III: a history of the controversy. *Archives of General Psychiatry* **42**, 187–96.

Beck AT, Emery G and Greenberg RL (1985). *Anxiety Disorders and Phobias: A Cognitive Perspective*. New York: Basic.

Bedford A, Foulds GA and Sheffield BF (1977). A new personal disturbance scale (DSSI/SAD). *British Journal of Social and Clinical Psychology* **15**, 387–94.

Benaim S, Horder J and Anderson J (1973). Hysterical epidemic in a classroom. *Psychological Medicine* **30**, 366–73.

Bialos D, Giller E, Jatlow P, Docherty J and Harkness MSW (1982). Recurrence of depression after long-term amitriptyline treatment. *American Journal of Psychiatry* **139**, 325–7.

Bianchi GN (1973). Patterns of hypochondriasis: a principal components analysis. *British Journal of Psychiatry* **122**, 541–8.

Bielski RJ and Friedel RO (1976). Prediction of tricyclic anti-depressant response: a critical review. *Archives of General Psychiatry* **33**, 1479–89.

Bishop ER Jr (1980). Monosymptomatic hypochondriasis. *Psychosomatics* **21**, 731–47.

Blackburn IM, Bishop S, Glen AIM, Whalley JJ and Christie JE (1981). The efficacy of cognitive therapy in depression: a treatment trial using cognitive therapy and pharmacotherapy, each alone and in combination. *British Journal of Psychiatry* **139**, 181–9.

Blanchard EB, Gerardi RJ, Kolb LC and Barlow DH (1986). The utility of the Anxiety Disorders Interview Schedule (ADIS) in the diagnosis of post-traumatic stress disorder (PTSD) in Vietnam veterans. *Behaviour Research and Therapy* **24**, 577–81.

Bonn JA, Harrison J and Rees W (1971). Lactate-induced anxiety: therapeutic application. *British Journal of Psychiatry* **119**, 468–70.

Boyd JH (1986). Use of mental health services for the treatment of panic disorder. *American Journal of Psychiatry* **143**, 1569–74.

Boyd JH, Burke JD, Gruenberg E, Holzer CE III, Rae DS et al. (1984). Exclusion criteria of DSM-III: a study of co-occurrence of hierarchy-free syndromes. *Archives of General Psychiatry* **41**, 983–9.

Brantigan CO, Brantigan TA and Joseph N (1982). Effect of beta-blockade and beta stimulation on stage fright. *American Journal of Medicine* **72**, 88–94.

Breier A, Charney DS and Heninger GR (1984). Major depression in patients with agoraphobia and panic disorder. *Archives of General Psychiatry* **41**, 1129–35.

Breier A, Charney DS and Heninger GR (1985). The diagnostic validity of anxiety disorders and their relationship to depressive illness. *American Journal of Psychiatry* **142**, 787–97.

Breier A, Charney DS and Heninger GR (1986). Agoraphobia with panic attacks: development, diagnostic stability and course of illness. *Archives of General Psychiatry* **43**, 1029–36.

Breuer J and Freud S (1983). On the psychical mechanism of hysterical phenomena: preliminary communication. In: *Complete Psychological Works*, Vol. 2 (trans. J Strachey, 1955), pp. 1–17. London: Hogarth Press.

Briquet P (1859). *Traite Clinique et Therapeutique de l'Hysterie* Paris: Baillière.

Brown F (1936). The bodily complaint: a study of hypochondriasis. *Journal of Mental Science* **82**, 295–359.

Buigues J and Vallejo J (1987). Therapeutic response to phenelzine in patients with panic disorder and agoraphobia with panic attacks. *Journal of Clinical Psychiatry* **48**, 55–9.

Butler G, Cullington A, Hibbert G, Klines I and Gelder M (1987). Anxiety management for persistent generalised anxiety. *British Journal of Psychiatry* **151**, 535–42.

Carroll BJ (1985). Dexamethasone suppression test: a review of contemporary confusion. *Journal of Clinical Psychiatry* **46**, 13–24.

Casey PR (1986). Psychiatric morbidity in general practice: a diagnostic approach, MD Thesis, University of Cork.

Casey P (1988). The epidemiology of personality disorder. In: *Personality Disorders: Diagnosis, Management and Course* (ed. P Tyrer), pp. 74–81. London: Wright.

Casey PR, Dillon S and Tyrer P (1984). The diagnostic status of patients with conspicuous psychiatric morbidity in primary care. *Psychological Medicine* **14**, 637–51.

Casey PR, Tyrer PJ and Platt S (1985). The relationship between social functioning and psychiatric symptomatology in primary care. *Social Psychiatry* **20**, 5–10.

Casey PR and Tyrer PJ (1986). Personality, functioning and symptomatology. *Journal of Psychiatric Research* **20**, 363–74.

Cassano GB, Perugi G, Maremmani I and Akiskal HS (1989). Social adjustment in dysthymia. In: *Dysthymic Disorder* (eds S Burton and HS Akiskal). London: Gaskell.

Charcot JM (1889). *Clinical Lectures on Diseases of the Nervous System*, Vol. 3 (trans. T Savill). London: New Sydenham Society.

Chodoff P (1972). The depressive personality: a critical review. *Archives of General Psychiatry* **27**, 666–73.

Chodoff P and Lyons H (1958). Hysteria, the hysterical personality and 'hysterical' conversion. *American Journal of Psychiatry* **114**, 734–40.

Chouinard G, Annable L, Fontaine R and Solyom L (1982). Alprazolam in the treatment of generalized anxiety and panic disorders: a double-blind placebo-controlled study. *Psychopharmacology* **77**, 229–33.

Clancy J, Noyes R, Hoenk PR and Slymen DJ (1978). Secondary depression in anxiety neurosis. *Journal of Nervous and Mental Disease* **166**, 846–50.

Clark DM (1986). A cognitive approach to panic. *Behaviour Research and Therapy* **24**, 461–70.

Clark DM, Salkovskis PN and Chalkley AJ (1985). Respiratory control as a treatment of panic attack. *Journal of Behaviour Therapy and Experimental Psychiatry* **16**, 23–30.

Cloninger CR (1987). Diagnosis of somatoform disorders: a critique of DSM-III. In: *Diagnosis and Classification in Psychiatry: a Critical Appraisal of DSM-III* (ed. G Tischler), pp. 243–59. Cambridge: Cambridge University Press.

Cloninger CR and Guze SB (1970). Psychiatric illness and female criminality: the role of sociopathy and hysteria in the antisocial women. *American Journal of Psychiatry* **127**, 303–11.

Cloninger CR and Guze SB (1975). Hysteria and parental psychiatric illness. *Psychological Medicine* **5**, 27–31.

Cloninger CR, Martin RL, Clayton P and Guze SB (1981). A blind follow-up and family study of anxiety neurosis: preliminary analysis of the St Louis 500. In: *Anxiety: New Research and Changing Concepts* (eds DF Klein and J Rabkin). New York: Raven Press.

Cloninger CR, Sigvardsson S, von Knorring A-L et al. (1984). An adoption study of somatoform disorders, II: identification of two discrete somatoform disorders. *Archives of General Psychiatry* **41**, 863–71.

Cooper B (1965). A study of one hundred chronic psychiatric patients identified in general practice. *British Journal of Psychiatry* **111**, 595–605.

Coppen AL and Metcalfe H (1965). The effect of a depressive illness on MMPI scores. *British Journal of Psychiatry* **111**, 236–9.

Coryell WH, Noyes R Jr and Clancy J (1982). Excess mortality in panic disorder: a comparison with primary unipolar depression. *Archives of General Psychiatry* **39**, 701–03.

Covi L, Park LE, Lipman RS, Uhlenhuth EH and Rickels K (1974). Factors affecting withdrawal response to certain minor tranquilizers. In: *Drug Abuse: Social and Psychopharmacological Aspects* (eds J Cole and JR Wittenborn), pp. 93–108. Springfield, Ill.: Thomas.

Crisp AH and McGuiness B (1976). Jolly fat: relation between obesity and psychoneurosis in general population. *British Medical Journal* 1, 7–9.

Crowe MJ, Marks IM, Agras WS and Leitenberg H (1972). Time-limited desensitisation, implosion and shaping for phobia patients: a crossover study. *Behaviour Research and Therapy* **10**, 319–28.

Crowe RR, Noyes R Jr, Pauls DL and Slymen D (1983). A family study of panic disorder. *Archives of General Psychiatry* **40**, 1065–9.

Crowe RR, Noyes R Jr, Wilson AF, Elston RC and Ward LJ (1987). A linkage study of panic disorder. *Archives of General Psychiatry* **44**, 933–7.

Cutler B and Reed J (1975). Multiple personality – a single case study with a 15 year follow-up. *Psychological Medicine* **5**, 18–26.

Daly RJ (1983). Samuel Pepys and post-traumatic stress disorder. *British Journal of Psychiatry* **143**, 64–8.

Davidson J, Swartz M, Storck M, Krishnan RR and Hammett E (1985). A diagnostic and family study of post-traumatic stress disorder. *American Journal of Psychiatry* **142**, 90–3.

Dealy RS, Ishiki DM, Avery DH, Wilson LG and Dunner DL (1981). Secondary depression in anxiety disorders. *Comprehensive Psychiatry* **22**, 612–18.

DiNardo PA, O'Brien GT, Barlow DH, Waddell MT and Blanchard EB (1983). Reliability of DSM-III anxiety disorder categories using a new structured interview. *Archives of General Psychiatry* **40**, 1070–4.

Dundee JW and Pandit SK (1972). Anterograde amnesic effects of pethidine, hyoscine and diazepam in adults. *British Journal of Pharmacology* **44**, 140–4.

Dunn G (1983). Longitudinal records of anxiety and depression in general practice: the Second National Morbidity Survey. *Psychological Medicine* **13**, 897–906.

Emmelkamp PMG and Kuipers ACM (1979). Agoraphobia: a follow-up study 4 years after treatment. *British Journal of Psychiatry* **134**, 352–5.

Falloon IR, Lloyd GG and Harpin R (1981). The treatment of social phobia: real-life rehearsal with nonprofessional therapists. *Journal of Nervous and Mental Disease* **169**, 180–4.

Fawcett J and Kravitz HM (1983). Anxiety syndromes and their relationship to depressive illness. *Journal of Clinical Psychiatry* **44**, 8–11.

Feighner JP, Merideth CH and Hendrickson GA (1982). A double-blind comparison of buspirone and diazepam in outpatients with generalised anxiety disorder. *Journal of Clinical Psychiatry* **43** (Sect. 2), 103–7.

Fenton GW (1986). Epilepsy and hysteria. *British Journal of Psychiatry* **149**, 28–37.

Ferguson B and Tyrer P (1988). Classifying personality disorder. In: *Personality Disorders: Diagnosis, Management and Course* (ed. P Tyrer), pp. 12–32. London: Wright.

Fewtrell WD (1984). Relaxation and depersonalisation. *British Journal of Psychiatry* **145**, 217.

Figley CR (ed.) (1978). *Stress Disorders among Vietnam Veterans: Theory, Research, and Treatment*. New York: Brunner/Mazel.

Finlay-Jones R and Brown GW (1981). Types of stressful life events and the onset of anxiety and depressive disorders. *Psychological Medicine* **11**, 803–15.

Flicker DJ (1956). Malingering: a symptom. *Journal of Nervous and Mental Disease* **123**, 23–31.

Foa EB, Steketee G, Kozak MJ and Dugger D (1987). Imipramine and placebo in the treatment of obsessive–compulsives: their effect on depression and obsessional symptoms. *Psychopharmacology Bulletin* **23**, 8–11.

Fontaine R, Chouinard G and Annable L (1984). Rebound anxiety in anxious patients after abrupt withdrawal of benzodiazepine treatment. *American Journal of Psychiatry* **141**, 848–52.

Fordyce WE (1986). Learning processes in pain. In: *Psychology of Pain*, 2nd edn (ed. RA Sternbach) pp. 49–66. New York: Raven Press.

Foulds G (1976). *The Hierarchical Nature of Personal Illness*. London: Academic Press.

Frances A (1980). The DSM-III personality disorders section: a commentary. *American Journal of Psychiatry* **137**, 1050–4.

Frances A and Voss CB (1987). Dysthymic disorder complicated by bouts of major depression. *Hospital and Community Psychiatry* **38**, 461–3.

Fredman L, Weissman MM, Leaf PJ and Bruce ML (1988). Social functioning in community residents with depression and other psychiatric disorders: results of the New Haven Epidemiologic Catchment Area Study. *Journal of Affective Disorders* **15**, 103-13.

Freud S (1895a). On the grounds for detaching a particular syndrome from neurasthenia under the description 'anxiety neurosis'. In: *Complete Psychological Works*, Vol. 3 (trans. J Strachey, 1962), pp. 85–117. London: Hogarth Press.

Freud S (1895b). Obsessions and phobias: their physical mechanisms and their aetiology. In: *Complete Psychological Works*, Vol. 3 (trans. J Strachey, 1962), pp. 69–89. London: Hogarth Press.

Freud S (1908). Character and anal-eroticism. In: *Complete Psychological Works*, Vol. 9 (trans. J Strachey, 1959), pp. 167–75. London: Hogarth Press.

Freud S (1926). Inhibitions, symptoms and anxiety. In: *Complete Psychological Works*, Vol. 20 (trans. J Strachey, 1959), pp. 75–174. London: Hogarth Press.

Friedman K, Shear MK and Frances A (1985). DSM-III personality disorders in panic patients. *Journal of Personality Disorders* **2**, 132–6.

Fromm E (1942). *Fear of Freedom*. London: Routledge.

Fyer AJ (1989). Reliability of anxiety assessment II: symptom agreement. *Archives of General Psychiatry*. (in press)

Ganser S (1898). A peculiar hysterical state. *Archivs für Psychiatrie und Nervenkrankheit* **30**, 633–9 (trans. CE Schorer) *British Journal of Criminology* **5**, 120–6.

Gatfield PD and Guze SB (1962). Prognosis and differential diagnosis of conversion reactions (a follow-up study). *Diseases of the Nervous System* **23**, 1–8.

Gelder MG (1986). Panic attacks: new approaches to an old problem. *British Journal of Psychiatry* **149**: 346–52.

Gelder MG and Marks IM (1966). Severe agoraphobia: a controlled prospective trial of behaviour therapy. *British Journal of Pychiatry* **112**, 309–19.

Ghosh A and Marks IM (1987). Self-treatment of agoraphobia by exposure. *Behavioural Therapy* **18**, 3–16.

Gittelman R and Klein DF (1984). Relationship between separation anxiety and panic and agoraphobic disorders. *Psychopathology* **17** (Suppl. 1), 56–65.

Gittleson NL (1966). The effects of obsessions on depressive psychosis. *British Journal of Psychiatry* **112** 253–8.

Goldstein SG and Linden JD (1969). Multivariate classification of alcoholics by means of the MMPI. *Journal of Abnormal Psychology* **74**, 661–9.

Gorman JM and Gorman LK (1987). Drug treatment of social phobia. *Journal of Affective Disorders* **13**, 183–92.

Granville-Grossman KL and Turner P (1966). The effect of propranolol on anxiety. *Lancet* i, 788–90.

Green BL, Grace MC, Lindy JD, Titchener JL and Lindy JG (1983). Levels of functional impairment following a civilian disaster: the Beverly Hills Supper Club fire. *Journal of Consulting and Clinical Psychology* **51**, 573–80.

Greenblatt DJ and Shader RI (1974). *Benzodiazepines in Clinical Practice*. New York: Raven Press.

Gregory S, Shawcross CR and Gill D (1985). The Nottingham ECT study: a double-blind comparison of bilateral, unilateral and simulated ECT in

172    *CLASSIFICATION OF NEUROSIS*

depressive illness (Mapperley Hospital, Nottingham). *British Journal of Psychiatry* **146**, 520–4.

Griez E and Van den Hout MA (1986). $CO_2$ inhalation in the treatment of panic attacks. *Behavior Research and Therapy* **24**, 145–50.

Grimshaw L (1964). Obsessional disorder and neurological illness. *Journal of Neurology, Neurosurgery and Psychiatry* **27**, 229–31.

Grinker RR and Spiegel JP (1943). *War Neurosis in North Africa: The Tunisian Campaign, January to May 1943.* New York: Josiah Macy Jr Foundation.

Gruenberg EM (1969). How can the new diagnostic manual help? *International Journal of Psychiatry* **7**, 368–74.

Gunderson JG and Singer MT (1975). Defining borderline patients: an overview. *American Journal of Psychiatry* **132**, 1–10.

Gunderson JG and Elliott G (1985). The interface between borderline personality disorder and affective disorder. *American Journal of Psychiatry* **142**, 277–88.

Gurney C, Roth M, Garside RF, Kerr TA and Schapira K (1972). Studies in the classification of affective disorders: the relationship between anxiety states and depressive illnesses. II. *British Journal of Psychiatry* **121**, 162–6.

Guze SB (1967). The diagnosis of hysteria: what are we trying to do? *American Journal of Psychiatry* **123**, 491–8.

Guze SB (1970). The role of follow-up studies: their contribution to diagnostic classification as applied to hysteria. *Seminars in Psychiatry* **2**, 392–402.

Guze SB, Woodruff RA and Clayton PJ (1971a). Hysteria and antisocial personality: further evidence of an association. *American Journal of Psychiatry* **127**, 957–60.

Guze SB, Woodruff RA and Clayton PJ (1971b). A study of conversion symptoms in psychiatric out-patients. *American Journal of Psychiatry* **128**, 643–6.

Guze SB, Woodruff RA and Clayton PJ (1972). Sex, age and the diagnosis of hysteria (Briquet's syndrome). *American Journal of Psychiatry* **129**, 745–8.

Guze SB, Cloninger CR, Martin RL and Clayton PJ (1986). A follow-up and family study of Briquet's syndrome. *British Journal of Psychiatry* **149**, 17–23.

Hafner J and Milton F (1977). The influence of propranolol on the exposure *in vivo* of agoraphobics. *Psychological Medicine* **7**, 419–25.

Hallam RS (1978). Agoraphobia: a critical review of the concept. *British Journal of Psychiatry* **133**, 314–19.

Hallstrom C (1988). Studies of benzodiazepines: pharmacokinetics, efficacy and dependence. MD Thesis, University of Liverpool.

Hartley LR, Ungaden S, Davie I and Spencer DJ (1983). The effect of beta adrenergic blocking drugs on speakers' performance and memory. *British Journal of Psychiatry* **142**, 512.

Hecker E (1893). Über larvirte und abortive Angstzustande bei Neurasthenie. *Zentralblatt für Nervenheilkunde und Psychiatrie (Berlin)* **133**, 565–72.

Heninger GR and Charney DS (1987). Mechanism of action of antidepressant treatments: implications for the etiology and treatment of depressive disorders. In: *Psychopharmacology: The Third Generation of Progress* (ed. HY Meltzer), pp. 535–44. New York: Raven Press.

Hoehn-Saric R (1981). Characteristics of chronic anxiety patients. In: *Anxiety: New Research and Changing Concepts* (eds DF Klein and JG Rabkin), pp. 399–409. New York: Raven Press.

Hoehn-Saric R (1982a). Comparison of generalized anxiety disorder with panic disorder patients. *Psychopharmacological Bulletin* **18**, 104–8.

Hoehn-Saric R (1982b). Neurotransmitters in anxiety. *Archives of General Psychiatry* **39**, 735–42.

Hoehn-Saric R and McLeod DR (1985). Generalized anxiety disorder. *Psychiatric Clinics of North America* **8**, 73–88.

Horney K (1939). *New Ways in Psycho-analysis*. London: Kegan Paul.

Horowitz M (1986). *Stress Response Syndromes*, 2nd edn. New York: Jason Aronson.

Hyler SE and Spitzer RL (1978). Hysteria split asunder. *American Journal of Psychiatry* **135**, 1500–4.

Insel TR and Mueller EA (1984). The psychopharmacologic treatment of obsessive–compulsive disorder. In: *New Findings in Obsessive–Compulsive Disorder* (ed. TR Insel). Washington DC: American Psychiatric Press.

Insel TR and Johar J (1987). Psychopharmacologic approaches to obsessive–compulsive disorder. In: *Psychopharmacology: The Third Generation of Progress* (ed. HY Meltzer), pp. 1205–10. New York: Raven Press.

Jablensky A (1985). Approaches to the definition and classification of anxiety and related disorders in European psychiatry. In: *Anxiety and the Anxiety Disorders* (eds AH Tuma and JD Maser). Hillsdale, NJ: Erlbaum.

James IM, Pearson RM, Griffith DNW and Newbury P (1977). The effect of oxprenolol on stage fright in musicians. *Lancet ii*, 952.

Janet P (1894). *L'État Mental des Hysteriques*. Paris: Rueff.

Janet P (1903). *Les Obsessions et la Psychasthenie* (2 vols). Paris: Felix Alcan.

Jannoun L, Munby M, Catalan J and Gelder M (1980). A home-based treatment program for agoraphobia: replication and controlled evaluation. *Behavior Therapy* **11**, 294–305.

Jardine R, Martin NG and Henderson AS (1984). Genetic covariation between neuroticism and the symptoms of anxiety and depression. *Genetic Epidemiology* **1**, 89–107.

Jellinek EM (1960).*The Disease Concept of Alcoholism*. New Brunswick, NJ: Hillhouse Press.

Jenike MA (1981). Rapid response of severe obsessive–compulsive disorder to tranylcypromine. *American Journal of Psychiatry* **138**, 1249–51.

Johnston D and Gath D (1973). Arousal levels and attribution effects in diazepam-assisted flooding. *British Journal of Psychiatry* **222**, 463–6.

Johnstone EC, Cunningham Owens DG, Frith CD, McPherson K, Dowie C et al. (1980). Neurotic illness and its response to anxiolytic and antidepressant treatment. *Psychological Medicine* **10**, 321–8.

Jung CG (1954). Medicine and psychotherapy. In: *Collected Works 16: Essays on the Psychology of the Transference and Other Subjects* (trans. RFC Hull). London: Routledge and Kegan Paul.

Kahn RJ, McNair DM, Lipman RS, Covi L, Rickels K et al. (1986). Imipramine and chlordiazepoxide in depressive and anxiety disorders: II. efficacy in anxious out-patients. *Archives of General Psychiatry* **43**, 79–85.

Kardiner A (1941). *The Traumatic Neuroses of War.* New York: Hoeber.

Katon W, Vitaliano PP, Russo J, Jones M and Anderson K (1987). Panic disorder: spectrum of severity and somatization. *Journal of Nervous and Mental Disease* **175**, 12–19.

Keller MB, Klerman GL, Lavori PW et al. (1982). Treatment received by depressed patients. *Journal of the American Medical Association* **248**, 1848–55.

Kelly D, Guirguis W, Frommer E, Mitchell-Heggs N and Sargant W (1970). Treatment of phobic states with antidepressants. *British Journal of Psychiatry* **116**, 387–98.

Kelly D, Mitchell-Heggs N and Sherman D (1971). Anxiety and the effects of sodium lactate assessed clinically and physiologically. *British Journal of Psychiatry* **119**, 129–41.

Kendell RE (1968). *The Classification of Depressive Illnesses.* London: Oxford University Press.

Kendell RE (1974). The stability of psychiatric diagnoses. *British Journal of Psychiatry* **124**, 352–6.

Kendell RE (1975). *The Role of Diagnosis in Psychiatry.* Oxford: Blackwell.

Kendell RE (1976). The classification of depressions: a review of contemporary confusion. *British Journal of Psychiatry* **129**, 15–28.

Kenyon FE (1965). Hypochondriasis: a survey of some historical, clinical and social aspects. *British Journal of Medical Psychology* **38**, 117–33.

Kerr TA, Roth M, Schapira K and Gurney C (1972). The assessment and prediction of outcome in affective disorders. *British Journal of Psychiatry* **121** 167–74.

Kiloh LG, Andrews G, Neilson M and Bianchi GN (1972). The relationship of the syndromes called endogenous and neurotic depression. *British Journal of Psychiatry* **121**, 183–96.

Kilpatrick DG, Best CL, Veronen LJ, Amick AE, Villeponteaux LA et al. (1985). Mental health correlates of criminal victimization: a random community survey. *Journal of Consulting and Clinical Psychology* **53**, 866–73.

King R, Margraf J, Ehlers A and Maddock R (1986). Panic disorder – overlap with symptoms of somatization disorder. In: *Panic and Phobias: Empirical Evidence of Theoretical Models and Longterm Effects of Behavioral Treatments* (eds I Hand and HU Wittchen). Berlin: Springer-Verlag.

Kinston W and Rosser R (1974). Disaster: effects on mental and physical state. *Journal of Psychosomatic Research* **18**, 437–56.

Klein DF (1964). Delineation of two drug-responsive anxiety syndromes. *Psychopharmacologia* **5**, 397–408.

Klein DF (1967). Importance of psychiatric diagnosis in prediction of clinical drug effects. *Archives of General Psychiatry* **16**, 118–25.

Klein DF (1981). Anxiety reconceptualized. In: *Anxiety: New Research and Changing Concepts* (ed. DF Klein and JG Rabkin), pp. 235–63. New York: Raven Press.

Klein DF and Fink M (1962). Psychiatric reaction patterns to imipramine. *American Journal of Psychiatry* **119**, 432–8.

Klein DF, Gittelman R, Quitkin F and Rifkin A (1980). *Diagnosis and Drug Treatment of Psychiatric Disorder: Adults and Children,* 2nd edn, p. 561.

Baltimore: Williams and Wilkins.

Klein DF and Klein H (1989a). The definition and psychopharmacology of spontaneous panic and phobia. In: *Psychopharmacology of Anxiety* (ed. P Tyrer), pp. 135–62. Oxford: Oxford University Press.

Klein DF and Klein H (1989b). The nosology, genetics, and theory of spontaneous panic and phobia. In: *Psychopharmacology of Anxiety* (ed. P Tyrer), pp. 163–95. Oxford: Oxford University Press.

Klerman GL (1988). Principles of interpersonal psychotherapy for depression. In: *Depression and Mania*. (eds A Georgotas and R Cancro), pp. 490–501. Amsterdam: Elsevier.

Klerman GL, Budman S, Berwick D, Weissman MM, Damico-White J *et al.* (1987). Efficacy of a brief psychosocial intervention for symptoms of stress and distress among patients in primary care. *Medical Care* **25**, 1078–88.

Koch JLA (1891). *Die psychopathischen Minderwertigkeiten.* Ravensburg: Dorn.

Kuch K, Swinson RP and Kirby M (1985). Post-traumatic stress disorder after car accidents. *Canadian Journal of Psychiatry* **30**, 426–7.

Lader MH (1967). Palmar skin conductance measures in anxiety and phobic states. *Journal of Psychosomatic Research* **11**, 271–81.

Lader M and Sartorius N (1968). Anxiety in patients with hysterical conversion symptoms. *Journal of Neurology, Neurosurgery and Psychiatry* **31**, 490–5.

Lader MH and Marks IM (1971). *Clinical Anxiety.* London: Heinemann.

Lader MH and Mathews A (1970). Physiological changes during spontaneous panic attacks. *Journal of Psychosomatic Research* **14**, 377–82.

*Lancet* (1982). Goodbye neurosis? *Lancet ii*, 29.

Lazare A, Klerman GL and Armor DJ (1966). Oral, obsessive and hysterical personality patterns. *Archives of General Psychiatry* **14**, 624–30.

Leckman JF, Merikangas KR, Pauls DL, Prusoff BA and Weissman MM (1983a). Anxiety disorders and depression: contradictions between family study data and DSM-III conventions. *American Journal of Psychiatry* **140**, 880–2.

Leckman JF, Weissman MM, Merikangas KR, Pauls DL and Prusoff BA (1983b). Panic disorder and major depression: increased risk of depression, alcoholism, panic, and phobic disorders in families of depressed probands with panic disorder. *Archives of General Psychiatry* **40**, 1055–60.

Leckman JF, Weissman MM, Merikangas KR, Pauls DL and Prusoff BA (1984). Methodologic differences in major depression and panic disorder studies. *Archives of General Psychiatry* **41**, 722–3.

Lee AS and Murray RM (1988). The long-term outcome of Maudsley depressives. *British Journal of Psychiatry* **153**, 741–51.

Leff JP (1978). Psychiatrists' versus patients' concepts of unpleasant emotions. *British Journal of Psychiatry* **133**, 306–13.

Lewis AJ (1934). Melancholia: a historical review. *Journal of Mental Science* **80**, 1–42.

Lewis A (1938). States of depression: their clinical and aetiological differentiation. *British Medical Journal 2*, 875–8.

Lewis AJ (1975). The survival of hysteria. *Psychological Medicine* **5**, 9–12.

Liebowitz MR (1985). Imipramine in the treatment of panic disorder and its complications. *Psychiatric Clinics of North America* **8**, 37–47.

Liebowitz MR, Fyer AJ, Gorman JM, Dillon D, Appleby IL *et al.* (1984a). Lactate provocation of panic attacks: I. Clinical and behavioral findings. *Archives of General Psychiatry* **41**, 764–70.

Liebowitz MR, Quitkin FM, Stewart JW, McGrath PJ, Harrison W *et al.* (1984b). Phenelzine v. imipramine in atypical depression: a preliminary report. *Archives of General Psychiatry* **41**, 669–77.

Liebowitz MR, Quitkin FM, Stewart JW, McGrath PJ, Harrison W *et al.* (1985a). Effect of panic attacks on the treatment of atypical depressives. *Psychopharmacology Bulletin* **21**, 558–61.

Liebowitz MR, Gorman JM, Fyer AJ and Klein DF (1985b). Social phobia: review of a neglected anxiety disorder. *Archives of General Psychiatry* **42**, 729–36.

Liebowitz MR, Fyer AJ, Gorman JM, Campeas RB, Sandberg DP *et al.* (1988). Tricyclic therapy of the DSM-III anxiety disorders: a review with implications for further research. *Journal of Psychiatric Research* **22** (Supp. 1), 7–31.

Lindemann E (1944). Symptomatology and management of acute grief. *American Journal of Psychiatry* **101**, 141–8.

Linden W (1981). Exposure treatments for focal phobias. *Archives of General Psychiatry* **38**, 769–75.

Lipman RS, Covi L, Rickels K, McNair DM, Downing R *et al.* (1986). Imipramine and chlordiazepoxide in depressive and anxiety disorders: I. Efficacy in depressed out-patients. *Archives of General Psychiatry* **43**, 68–77.

Lipsedge MS, Hajioff P, Huggins P, Napier L, Pearce J *et al.* (1973). The management of severe agoraphobia: a comparison of iproniazid and systemic desensitization. *Psychopharmacologia* **32**, 67–80.

Løberg T (1981). MMPI-based personality subtypes of alcoholics: relationships to drinking history, psychometrics and neuropsychological deficits. *Journal of Studies on Alcohol* **42**, 766–82.

Loranger AW, Susman VL, Oldham JM and Russakoff LM (1985). *Personality Disorder Examination (PDE). A Structured Interview for DSM-III-R and ICD-9 Personality Disorders*, WHO/ADAMHA pilot version. White Plains, NY: The New York Hospital, Cornell Medical Center, Westchester Division.

Lydiard RB and Ballenger JC (1987). Antidepressants in panic disorder and agoraphobia. *Journal of Affective Disorders* **13**, 153–68.

Mann AH, Jenkins R and Belsey E (1981a). The twelve-month outcome of patients with neurotic illness in general practice. *Psychological Medicine* **11**, 535–50.

Mann AH, Jenkins R, Cutting JC and Cowen PJ (1981b). The development and use of a standardized assessment of abnormal personality. *Psychological Medicine* **11**, 839–47.

Mapother E and Lewis A (1941). In: *A Textbook of the Practice of Medicine*, 6th edn (ed. FW Price), pp. 1807–60. London: Oxford University Press.

Margraf J, Taylor CB, Ehlers A, Roth WT and Agras WS (1987). Panic attacks in the natural environment. *Journal of Nervous and Mental Disease* **175**, 558–65.

Marks IM (1970). Agoraphobic syndrome (phobic anxiety state). *Archives of General Psychiatry* **23**, 538–53.

Marks IM (1971). Phobic disorders four years after treatment: a prospective follow-up. *British Journal of Psychiatry* **118**, 683–6.

Marks IM (1983). Are there anti-compulsive or anti-phobic drugs? Review of the evidence. *British Journal of Psychiatry* **140**, 338–47.

Marks IM (1987a). *Fears, Phobias and Rituals: Panic, Anxiety and their Disorders*. London: Oxford University Press.

Marks IM (1987b). Agoraphobia, panic disorder and related conditions in the DSM-III-R and ICD-10. *Journal of Psychopharmacology* **1**, 6–12.

Marks I (1987c). Classification of phobic and obsessive-compulsive phenomena. In: *Handbook of Anxiety* (eds R Noyes, M Roth and G Burrows). Amsterdam: Elsevier.

Marks IM, Hodgson, R and Rachman S (1975). Treatment of chronic obsessive–compulsive disorder two years after *in vivo* exposure. *British Journal of Psychiatry* **127**, 349–64.

Marks IM, Stern RS, Mawson D, Cobb J and McDonald R (1980). Clomipramine and exposure for obsessive–compulsive rituals. *British Journal of Psychiatry* **136**, 1–25.

Marks IM, Grey S, Cohen SD, Hill R, Mawson D et al. (1983). Imipramine and brief therapist-aided exposure in agoraphobics having self-exposure homework: a controlled trial. *Archives of General Psychiatry* **40**, 153–62.

Marks IM, Lelliott P, Basoglu M and Noshirvani H et al. (1988). Clomipramine self-exposure and therapist-aided exposure for compulsive rituals. *British Journal of Psychiatry* **152**, 522–34.

Marks I and O'Sullivan G (1989). Anti-anxiety drug and psychological treatment effects in agoraphobia/panic and obsessive–compulsive disorders. In: *Psychopharmacology of Anxiety* (ed. P Tyrer), pp. 196–242. Oxford: Oxford University Press.

Martin NG, Jardine R, Andrews G and Heath AC (1988). Anxiety disorders and neuroticism: are there genetic factors specific to panic? *Acta Psychiatrica Scandinavica* **77**, 698–706.

Martin RL, Cloninger CR and Guze SB (1979). The evaluation of diagnostic concordance in follow-up studies, II: a blind follow-up of female criminals. *Journal of Psychiatric Research* **15**, 107–25.

Mathews AM, Gelder MG and Johnston DW (1981). *Agoraphobia: Nature and Treatment*. Oxford: Oxford University Press.

Mavissakalian MR, Turner SM, Michelson L and Jacob R (1985). Tricyclic antidepressants in obsessive–compulsive disorder: anti-obsessional or antidepressant agents? *American Journal of Psychiatry* **142**, 572–6.

Mayou R (1976). The nature of bodily symptoms. *British Journal of Psychiatry* **129**, 55–60.

Mbatia J and Tyrer P (1988). Personality status of dangerous patients at a special hospital. In: *Personality Disorders: Diagnosis, Management and Course* (ed. P Tyrer), pp. 105–11. London: Wright.

Mears R and Horvath T (1972). Acute and chronic hysteria. *British Journal of Psychiatry* **121**, 653–7.

Medical Research Council (Brain Injuries Committee) (1941). *A Glossary of Psychological Terms Commonly Used in Cases of Head Injury*, War Memorandum No. 4, London: HMSO.

Medical Research Council (1965). Report to the Medical Council by its Clinical Psychiatry Committee. Clinical trial of the treatment of depressive illness. *British Medical Journal* 1, 881–6.

Mendels J, Weinstein N and Cochrane C (1972). The relationship between anxiety and depression. *Archives of General Psychiatry* 27, 649–53.

Merskey H (1979). *The Analysis of Hysteria*. London: Baillière Tindall.

Merskey H (1986). The importance of hysteria. *British Journal of Psychiatry* 149, 23–8.

Merskey H and Buhrich NA (1975). Hysteria and organic brain disease. *British Journal of Medical Psychology* 48, 359–66.

Miller H (1967). Depression. *British Medical Journal* 1, 257–62.

Millon T (1983). The DSM-III: an insider's perspective. *American Psychologist* 38, 804–14./

Montgomery SA and Åsberg M (1979). A new depression scale designed to be sensitive to change. *British Journal of Psychiatry* 134, 382–9.

Morris JB and Beck AT (1974). The efficacy of antidepressant drugs. A review of research (1958 to 1972). *Archives of General Psychiatry* 30, 667–74.

Moss PD and McEvedy CP (1966). An epidemic of overbreathing among schoolgirls. *British Medical Journal* 2, 1295–300.

Mountjoy CQ and Roth M (1982). Studies in the relationship between depressive disorders and anxiety states. Part 1. Rating scales. *Journal of Affective Disorders* 4, 127–47.

Mullaney JA and Trippett CJ (1979). Alcohol dependence and phobias: clinical description and relevance. *British Journal of Psychiatry* 135, 565–73.

Muller JJ, Chafetz ME and Blare HT (1967). Acute psychiatric services in the general hospital: III, statistical survey. *American Journal of Psychiatry* 124, (46), 56.

Munjack DJ and Moss HB (1981). Affective disorders and alcoholism in families of agoraphobics. *Archives of General Psychiatry* 38, 869–71.

Murphy GE, Simons AD, Wetzel RD and Lustmann PJ (1984a). Cognitive therapy and pharmacotherapy singly and together in the treatment of depression. *Archives of General Psychiatry* 41, 33–41.

Murphy SM, Owen RT and Tyrer PJ (1984b). Withdrawal symptoms after six weeks treatment with diazepam. *Lancet i*, 1389.

Myers JK, Weissman MM, Tischler GL, Holzer CE, Leaf PJ *et al.* (1984). Six month prevalence of psychiatric disorders in three communities, 1980–1982. *Archives of General Psychiatry* 41, 959–67.

Newman CJ (1976). Children of disaster: clinical observations at Buffalo Creek. *American Journal of Psychiatry* 133, 306–12.

Noble P and Lader M (1972). Physiological differences in depressive illness. *British Journal of Psychiatry* 121, 267–70.

Noyes RJ, Clancy J, Crowe R, Hoenk RP and Slymen DJ (1983). The familial prevalence of anxiety neurosis. *Archives of General Psychiatry* 35, 1067–74.

Noyes R Jr, Anderson DJ, Clancy J, Crowe RR, Slyman DJ *et al.* (1984). Diazepam and propranolol in panic disorder and agoraphobia. *Archives of General Psychiatry* 41, 287–92.

Noyes R, Reich J, Clancy J and O'Gorman TW (1986a). Reduction in hypochondriasis with treatment of panic disorder. *British Journal of Psychiatry* **149**, 631–5.

Noyes R Jr, Crowe RR, Harris EL, Hamra BJ, McChesney CM *et al.* (1986b). Relationship between panic disorder and agoraphobia: a family study. *Archives of General Psychiatry* **43**, 227–32.

Ost LG, Jerremalm A and Johansson J (1981). Individual response patterns and the effects of different behavioral methods in the treatment of social phobia. *Behaviour Research and Therapy* **19**, 1–16.

Paykel ES (1971). Classification of depressed patients: a cluster analysis derived grouping. *British Journal of Psychiatry* **118**, 275–88.

Paykel ES, Myers JK, Dienelt MN, Klerman GL, Lindenthal JJ *et al.* (1969). Life events and depression: a controlled study. *Archives of General Psychiatry* **21**, 753–60.

Paykel ES and Prusoff BA (1973). Relationships between personal dimensions: neuroticism and extraversion against obsessive, hysterical and oral personality. *British Journal of Social and Clinical Psychology* **12**, 309–18.

Paykel ES, Klerman GL and Prusoff BA (1976). Personality and symptom pattern in depression. *British Journal of Psychiatry* **129**, 327–34.

Paykel ES, Rowan PR, Parker RR and Bhat AV (1982). Response to phenelzine and amitriptyline in subtypes of out-patient depression. *Archives of General Psychiatry* **39**, 1041–9.

Paykel ES, Parker RR, Rowan PR, Rao BM and Taylor CN (1983). Nosology of atypical depression. *Psychological Medicine* **13**, 131–40.

Pecknold JC, Swinson RP, Kuch, K and Lewis LP (1988). Alprazolam in panic disorder and agoraphobia: results from a multicenter trial: III. Discontinuation effects. *Archives of General Psychiatry* **45**, 429–36.

Perley M and Guze SB (1962). Hysteria – the stability and usefulness of clinical criteria. *New England Journal of Medicine* **266**, 421–6.

Perse TL, Greist JH, Jefferson JW, Rosenfeldt R and Dar R (1987). Fluvoxamine treatment of obsessive–compulsive disorder. *American Journal of Psychiatry* **144**, 1543–8.

Pfohl B, Stangl D and Zimmerman M (1982). *Structured Interview for DSM-III Personality Disorders (SID–P)*. Iowa City: University of Iowa Hospitals and Clinics.

Pitts FN and McClure JN (1967). Lactate metabolism in anxiety neurosis. *New England Journal of Medicine* **277**, 1329–36.

Prince M (1905). *Dissociation of a Personality*, 2nd edn. London: Longmans Green.

Prusoff B and Klerman GL (1974). Differentiating depressed from anxious neurotic out-patients. *Archives of General Psychiatry* **30**, 302–9.

Quitkin FM, Rifkin A, Kaplan J and Klein DF (1972). Phobic anxiety syndrome complicated by drug dependence and addiction. *Archives of General Psychiatry* **27**, 159–62.

Rapoport J, Elkins R and Mikkelson E (1980). Chlorimipramine in adolescents with obsessive–compulsive disorder. *Psychopharmocology Bulletin* **16**, 61–3.

Raskin M, Peeke HVS, Dickman W and Pinsker H (1982). Panic and generalised anxiety disorder. *Archives of General Psychiatry* **39**, 687–9.

Ravaris CL, Nies A, Robinson DS, Ives JO and Bartlett D (1976). A multiple-dose controlled study of phenelzine in depressive–anxiety states. *Archives of General Psychiatry* **33**, 347–50.

Reed JL (1975). The diagnosis of 'hysteria'. *Psychological Medicine* **5**, 13–17.

Rice KM and Blanchard EB (1982). Biofeedback in the treatment of anxiety disorders. *Clinical Psychological Review* **2**, 557–77.

Rickels K, Weisman K, Norstad N, Singer M, Stoltz D et al. (1982). Buspirone and diazepam in anxiety: a controlled study. *Journal of Clinical Psychiatry* **43**, 81–6.

Riskind JH, Beck AT, Berchick RJ, Brown G and Steer RA (1987). Reliability of DSM-III diagnoses for major depression and generalized anxiety using the structured clinical interview for DSM-III. *Archives of General Psychiatry* **44**, 817–20.

Robins LN, Helzer JE, Weissman MM, Orvaschel H et al. (1984). Life-time prevalence of specific psychiatric disorders at three sites. *Archives of General Psychiatry* **41**, 949–58.

Robins LN, Wing J, Wittchen H-U, Helzer JE et al. (1988). The Composite International Diagnostic Interview: an epidemiologic instrument suitable for use in conjunction with different diagnostic systems and in different cultures. *Archives of General Psychiatry* **45**, 1069–77.

Robinson DS, Nies A, Ravaris CL, Ives JO and Bartlett D (1978). Clinical pharmacology of phenelzine. *Archives of General Psychiatry* **35**, 629–35.

Rosenberg CM (1968). Complications of obsessional neurosis. *British Journal of Psychiatry* **114**, 477–78.

Roth M (1959). The phobic anxiety–depersonalization syndrome. *Proceedings of the Royal Society of Medicine* **52**, 587–96.

Roth M, Gurney C, Garside RF and Kerr TA (1972). Studies in the classification of affective disorders: the relationship between anxiety states and depressive illnesses. I. *British Journal of Psychiatry* **121**, 147–61.

Roth M and Mountjoy CQ (1982). The distinction between anxiety states and depressive disorders. In: *Handbook of Affective Disorders* (ed. ES Paykel). Edinburgh: Churchill Livingstone.

Roth M, Mountjoy CQ and Caetano D (1982). Further investigations into the relationship between depressive disorders and anxiety states. *Pharmacopsychiatry* **15**, 135–41.

Rush AJ, Beck AT, Kovacs M and Hollon SD (1977). Comparative efficacy of cognitive therapy and pharmacotherapy in the treatment of depressed out-patients. *Cognitive Research and Therapy* **1**, 17–37.

Rutter ML (1987). Temperament, personality and personality disorder. *British Journal of Psychiatry* **150**, 443–58.

Salkovskis PM, Jones DRO and Clark DM (1985). Respiratory control in the treatment of panic attack: application and extension with concurrent measurement of behaviour and $pCO_2$. *British Journal of Psychiatry* **148**, 526–32.

Sargant W (1957). *Battle for the Mind. A Physiology of Conversion and Brain-Washing*. London: Heinemann.

Sargant W and Shorvon HJ (1945). Acute war neurosis. *Archives of Neurology and Psychiatry* **54**, 231–40.

Schapira K, Roth M, Kerr TA and Gurney C (1972). The prognosis of affective disorders: the differentiation of anxiety states from depressive illnesses. *British Journal of Psychiatry* 121, 175–81.

Seivewright N (1987). Relationship between life events and personality in psychiatric disorder. *Stress Medicine* 3, 163–8.

Seivewright N (1988). Personality disorder, life events and the onset of mental illness. In: *Personality Disorders: Diagnosis, Management and Course* (ed. P Tyrer), pp. 82–92. London: Wright.

Seivewright N and Tyrer P (1989). Relationship of dysthymia to anxiety and other neurotic disorders. in: *Dysthymic Disorder: A New Concept in Chronic Minor Depression* (eds S Burton and HS Akiskal). London: Gaskell. (in press)

Shapiro AK, Streuning EL, Shapiro E and Milcarek B (1983). Diazepam: how much better than placebo? *Journal of Psychiatric Research* 17, 51–73.

Sheehan DV (1983). *The Anxiety Disease.* New York: Charles Scribner's Sons.

Sheehan DV (1987). Benzodiazepines in panic disorder and agoraphobia. *Journal of Affective Disorders* 13, 169–81.

Sheehan DV, Ballenger J and Jacobsen G (1980). Treatment of endogenous anxiety with phobic, hysterical, and hypochondriacal symptoms. *Archives of General Psychiatry* 37, 51–9.

Sheehan DV and Sheehan KH (1983). The classification of phobic disorders. *International Journal of Psychiatric Medicine* 12, 243–66.

Sheehan DV, Coleman JH, Greenblatt DJ, Jones KJ, Levine PH *et al.* (1984). Some biochemical correlates of panic attacks with agoraphobic and their response to a new treatment. *Journal of Clinical Psychopharmacology* 4, 66–75.

Shehi M and Patterson W (1984). Treatment of panic with alprazolam and propranolol. *American Journal of Psychiatry* 141, 900–1.

Shepherd M, Cooper B, Brown AC and Kalton GW (1966). *Psychiatric Illness in General Practice.* Oxford: Oxford University Press.

Slater E (1943). The neurotic constitution: a statistical study of 2000 neurotic soldiers. *Journal of Neurology and Psychiatry* 6, 1–16.

Slater E (1965). Diagnosis of hysteria. *British Medical Journal 1*, 1395–9.

Slater, ETO and Glithero, E. (1965). A follow-up of patients diagnosed as suffering from 'hysteria'. *Journal of Psychosomatic Research* 9, 9–14.

Slater E and Shields J (1969). Genetical aspects of anxiety. *British Journal of Psychiatry* 3 (special publication), 62–71.

Smail P, Stockwell T, Canter S and Hodgson R (1984). Alcohol dependence and phobic anxiety states: I. A prevalence study. *British Journal of Psychiatry* 144, 53–7.

Smith GR, Markham W, Monson RA and Ray DC (1986). Psychiatric consultation in somatization disorder: a randomized controlled study. *New England Journal of Medicine* 314, 1407–13.

Snaith RP (1981). *Clinical Neurosis.* Oxford: Oxford University Press.

Solyom K, Heseltine GF, McClure DJ, Solyom C, Ledwidge B *et al.* (1973). Behavior therapy versus drug therapy in the treatment of phobic neurosis. *Canadian Psychiatric Association Journal* 18, 25–31.

Spitzer R and Endicott J (1983). *Schedule for Affective Disorders and Schizophrenia (SADS)*. New York: New York State Psychiatric Institute.

Spitzer R, Williams JBW and Gibbon M (1987). *Structured Interview for DSM-III-R Personality Disorders*. New York: Biometrics Research Department, New York State Psychiatric Institute.

Stangl D, Pfohl B, Zimmerman M, Bowers W and Carenthal C (1985). Structured interview for DSM-III personality disorders. *Archives of General Psychiatry* **42**, 591–6.

Stavrakaki C and Vargo B (1986). The relationship of anxiety and depression: a review of the literature. *British Journal of Psychiatry* **149**, 7–16.

Taylor SJ and Chave S (1964). *Mental Health and Environment*. London: Longman.

Teasdale JD (1985). Psychological treatments for depression: how do they work? *Behaviour Research and Therapy* **23**, 157–65.

Teasdale JD, Fennell MJV, Hibbert GA and Amies PL (1984). Cognitive therapy for major depressive disorder in primary care. *British Journal of Psychiatry* **144**, 400–6.

Telch MJ, Tearnan BH and Taylor CB (1983). Antidepressant medication in the treatment of agoraphobia: a critical review. *Behaviour Research and Therapy* **21**, 505–17.

Thigpen CH and Cleckley HM (1954). A case of multiple personality. *Journal of Abnormal and Social Psychology* **49**, 135–51.

Thoren P, Asberg M, Cronholm B, Jornestedt L and Traskman L (1980). Clomipramine treatment of obsessive–compulsive disorder: a controlled clinical trial. *Archives of General Psychiatry* **37**, 1281–9.

Thyer BA, Himle J, Curtis GC, Cameron OG and Nesse RM (1985). A comparison of panic disorder and agoraphobia with panic attacks. *Comprehensive Psychiatry* **26**, 208–14.

Thyer BA, Nesse RM, Curtis GC and Cameron OG (1986). Panic disorder: a test of the separation anxiety hypothesis. *Behaviour Research and Therapy* **24**, 209–11.

Thyer BA and Himle J (1987). Phobic anxiety and panic anxiety: how do they differ? *Journal of Anxiety Disorders* **1**, 59–67.

Torgersen S (1983). Genetic factors in anxiety disorders. *Archives of General Psychiatry* **40**, 1085–9.

Tyrer P (1973). Relevance of bodily feelings in emotion. *Lancet i*, 915–6.

Tyrer P (1976). *The Role of Bodily Feelings in Anxiety*. London: Oxford University Press.

Tyrer P (1979). Clinical use of monoamine oxidase inhibitors. In: *Psychopharmacology of Affective Disorders* (eds ES Paykel and A Coppen), pp. 159–78. Oxford: Oxford University Press.

Tyrer P (1982). Anxiety states. In: *Handbook of Affective Disorders* (ed. ES Paykel), pp. 59–69. London: Academic Press.

Tyrer P (1984a). Classification of anxiety. *British Journal of Psychiatry* **144**, 78–83.

Tyrer P (1984b). Clinical effects of abrupt withdrawal from tricyclic antidepressants and monoamine oxidase inhibitors. *Journal of Affective Disorders* **6**, 1–7.

Tyrer P (1985). Neurosis divisible? *Lancet i,* 685–8.

Tyrer P (1986a). New rows of neuroses – are they an illusion? *Integrative Psychiatry* **4**, 25–31.

Tyrer P (1986b). Classification of anxiety disorders: a critique of DSM-III. *Journal of Affective Disorders* **11**, 99–104.

Tyrer P (1988) Current status of beta-blocking drugs in the treatment of anxiety disorders. *Drugs* **36**, 773–83.

Tyrer P (1989) Choice of treatment in anxiety. In: *Psychopharmacology of Anxiety* (ed. P. Tyrer), pp. 255–82. Oxford: Oxford University Press.

Tyrer P, Candy J and Kelly DA (1973). A study of the clinical effects of phenelzine and placebo in the treatment of phobic anxiety. *Psychopharmacologia* **32**, 237–54.

Tyrer P and Steinberg D (1975). Symptomatic treatment of agoraphobia and social phobias: a follow-up study. *British Journal of Psychiatry* **127**, 163–8.

Tyrer P and Alexander J (1979). Classification of personality disorder. *British Journal of Psychiatry* **135**, 163–7.

Tyrer P, Gardner M, Lambourn J and Whitford M (1980a). Clinical and pharmacokinetic factors affecting response to phenelzine. *British Journal of Psychiatry* **136**, 359–65.

Tyrer P, Lee I and Alexander J (1980b). Awareness of cardiac function in anxious, phobic and hypochondriacal patients. *Psychological Medicine* **10**, 171–4.

Tyrer P, Casey P and Gall J (1983). The relationship between neurosis and personality disorder. *British Journal of Psychiatry* **142**, 404–8.

Tyrer P, Owen RT and Cicchetti DV (1984). The brief scale for anxiety: a subdivision of the comprehensive psychopathological rating scale. *Journal of Neurology, Neurosurgery and Psychiatry* **47**, 970–5.

Tyrer P, Casey PR and Seivewright N (1986). Common personality features in neurotic disorder. *British Journal of Medical Psychology* **59**, 289–94.

Tyrer P and Murphy S (1987). The place of benzodiazepines in psychiatric practice. *British Journal of Psychiatry* **151**, 719–23.

Tyrer P, Alexander J, Remington M and Riley P (1987a). Relationship between neurotic symptoms and neurotic diagnosis: a longitudinal study. *Journal of Affective Disorders* **13**, 13–21.

Tyrer P, Remington M and Alexander J (1987b). The outcome of neurotic disorders after out-patient and day hospital care. *British Journal of Psychiatry* **151**, 57–62.

Tyrer P and Alexander J (1988). Personality Assessment Schedule. In: *Personality Disorders: Diagnosis, Management and Course* (ed. P Tyrer), pp. 43–62. London: Wright.

Tyrer P and Shawcross C (1988). Monoamine oxidase inhibitors in anxiety disorders. *Journal of Psychiatric Research* **22** (Suppl. 1), 87–98.

Tyrer P, Casey P and Ferguson B (1988a). Personality disorder and mental illness. In: *Personality Disorders: Diagnosis, Management and Course* (ed. P Tyrer), pp. 93–104. London: Wright.

Tyrer P, Seivewright N, Murphy S, Ferguson B, Kingdon D *et al.* (1988b). The Nottingham study of neurotic disorder: comparison of drug and psychological treatments. *Lancet ii*, 235–40.

Uhde TW, Boulenger J-P, Roy-Byrne PP, Geraci MF, Vittone BJ et al. (1985). Longitudinal course of panic disorder: clinical and biological considerations: *Progress in Neuropsychopharmacology and Biological Psychiatry* **9**, 39–51.

Uhlenhuth EH, Balter MB, Mellinger GD, Cisin IH and Clinthrone J (1983). Symptom checklist syndromes in the general population: correlations with psychotherapeutic drug use. *Archives of General Psychiatry* **40**, 1167–73.

Ullrich R, Ullrich C, Crombach G and Peikert V (1975). Three flooding procedures for agoraphobia. In: *Progress in Behavior Therapy* (ed. JC Brengelmann), pp. 59–67. New York: Springer-Verlag.

Van der Kolk BA (1987). The drug treatment of post-traumatic stress disorder. *Journal of Affective Disorders* **13**, 203–13.

Van der Molen GM, Van den Hout MA, Van Dieren AC and Griez E (1989). Childhood separation anxiety: no specific precursor to panic disorders. *Journal of Anxiety Disorders*. (in press)

Van Valkenburg C, Akiskal HS, Puzantian V and Rosenthal T (1984). Anxious depressions: clinical, family history, and naturalistic outcome. Comparisons with panic and major depressive disorders. *Journal of Affective Disorders* **6**, 67–82.

Waddell MT, Barlow DH and O'Brien GT (1984). Cognitive and relaxation treatment for panic disorders: effects on panic versus 'background' anxiety. *Behaviour Research and Therapy* **22**, 393–402.

Walker L (1959). The prognosis for affective illness with overt anxiety. *Journal of Neurology, Neurosurgery and Psychiatry* **22**, 338–41.

Watson JP, Gaind R and Marks IM (1971). Prolonged exposure – a rapid treatment for phobias. *British Medical Journal 1*, 13–15.

Weissman MM, Kasl SV and Klerman GL (1976). Follow-up of depressed women after maintenance treatment. *American Journal of Psychiatry*, **133**, 757–60.

Weissman MM and Klerman GL (1977). The chronic depressive in the community: unrecognised and poorly treated. *Comprehensive Psychiatry* **18**, 523–32.

Weissman MM, Myers, JK and Harding PS (1978). Psychiatric disorder in a US urban community. *American Journal of Psychiatry* **135**, 459–62.

Weissman MM, Leaf PJ, Blazer DG, Boyd JH and Florio L (1986). The relationship between panic disorder and agoraphobia: an epidemiologic perspective. *Psychopharmacology Bulletin* **43**, 787–91.

Weissman MM, Jarrett RB and Rush JA (1987). Psychotherapy and its relevance to the pharmacotherapy of major depression: a decade later (1976–1985). In: *Psychopharmacology: The Third Generation of Progress* (ed. HY Meltzer), pp. 1059–70. New York: Raven Press.

West ED and Dally PJ (1959). Effects of iproniazid in depressive syndromes. *British Medical Journal 1*, 1491–4.

Westphal C (1871). Die agoraphobia: eine neuropathische Eischeinung. *Archives für Psychiatrie und Nervenkrankheiten* **3**, 384–412.

Whitlock FA (1967a). The Ganser syndrome. *British Journal of Psychiatry* **113**, 19–30.
Whitlock FA (1967b). The aetiology of hysteria. *Acta Psychiatrica Scandinavica* **43**, 144–62.
Wing JK, Cooper JE and Sartorius N (1974). *The Measurement and Classification of Psychiatric Symptoms*. Cambridge: Cambridge University Press.
Winokur G (1987). Family (genetic) studies in neurotic depression. *Journal of Psychiatric Research* **21**, 357–63.
Woodruff RA Jr, Guze SB and Clayton PJ (1971). Hysteria: studies of diagnosis outcome and prevalence. *Journal of the American Medical Association* **215**, 425–8.
World Health Organization (1978). *Mental Disorders: Glossary and Guide to their Classification in Accordance with the Ninth Revision of the International Classification of Diseases*. Geneva: World Health Organization.
World Health Organization (1988). *International Classification of Diseases, Draft for Tenth Revision*, Geneva: World Health Organization.
Young JPR, Fenton GW and Lader MH (1971). Inheritance of neurotic traits: a twin study of the Middlesex Hospital Questionnaire. *British Journal of Psychiatry* **119**, 393–8.
Zigmond AS and Snaith RP (1983). The Hospital Anxiety and Depression Scale. *Acta Psychiatrica Scandinavica* **57**, 361–70.
Zitrin CM, Klein DF and Woerner MG (1978). Behavior therapy , supportive psychotherapy, imipramine, and phobias. *Archives of General Psychiatry* **35**, 307–16.
Zitrin CM, Klein DF, Woerner MG and Ross DC (1983). Treatment of phobias: I. Comparison of imipramine hydrochloride and placebo. *Archives of General Psychiatry* **40**, 125–38.

# Index

abreaction 90
acute stress reactions 118–9, 120,
    122, 129–30
adjustment disorders
    case history 119
    description 118–21
    differential diagnosis 127–28
    outcome 129–30
    stability 142
    treatment 130–31
affective disorders
    classification 63–4
affective personality disorder 63,
    70
agitation
    in depressive disorder 65–7
agoraphobia with panic disorder
    case history 44–5
    classification 43, 134
    development 32–3
    distinction from panic
        disorder 52
    drug treatment 56–62
    epidemiology 57
    exposure treatment 56–9
    mortality 35
    outcome 55–6
    overlap 54, 62
    reliability 28

    treatment 37
agoraphobia without panic disorder
    definition 43
    epidemiology 48
    overlap 52, 54
    treatment 56–9
AIDS phobia 42–3
alcohol dependence
    in panic disorder 35
    in post-traumatic stress
        disorder 129–30
    in social phobia 45–6
alprazolam
    in agoraphobia with panic 60
    dependence 58, 60
    in panic disorder 39, 56
    and personality disorder 35
    relapse after treatment 58
ambulatory depression 71
amitriptyline
    in obsessive–compulsive
        disorder 60
amnesia, see psychogenic amnesia
anankastic personality disorder
    classification 8
    in general neurotic
        syndrome 156–60
    and obsessive–compulsive
        disorder 54, 149

anniversary reactions 125
anorexia
    in depressive disorders 65–8, 71,
        151
anorexia nervosa 4–5, 50
anticipatory anxiety 36
antidepressents, *see also under
    individual drug names*
    in agoraphobia with panic 56–61
    dependence 58
    in depressive disorders 80–6
    in generalized anxiety
        disorder 39, 146
    in major depressive episode 146
    mechanism of action 57–8
    in obsessive–compulsive
        disorder 58
    in panic disorder 37–9
    in phobic disorder 57–8
antisocial personality disorder
    classification 9
    in neuroses 149
    somatization 115
    synonyms 17
anxiety attacks, *see* panic
anxiety disorders
    and adjustment disorders 122
    classification 2
    genetic aspects 160–2
    and personality disorder 151
    prognosis 78–9
    separation from depressive
        disorders 136–7
anxiety management training 25,
    85
anxiety neurosis 17–18, 63, 78–9,
    *see also* generalized anxiety
    disorder
    *and* panic disorder
anxiety–depressive (mixed)
    disorder, *see also* general
    neurotic syndrome
    classification 2, 140, 150–3, 163–4
    description 73
    outcome 75–6
    in stress and adjustment
        disorders 123–4
    validity 80, 148

anxious avoidant disorders 55, 61,
    151
anxious personality disorder 9, 10,
    29, 159
apprehension
    in generalized anxiety
        disorder 27
atypical depression 84
autoimmune disorders 114
autonomic symptoms 136–7
avoidance
    in agoraphobia 48, 151
    in classification of phobic
        disorder 43
    in general neurotic
        syndrome 156
    in post-traumatic stress
        disorder 124–5, 130
    in simple phobia 53
    in social phobia 53
avoidant personality disorder 9, 54

behaviour therapy, *see also*
    exposure therapies
    in adjustment disorders 130
    and cognitive therapy 82–4
*belle indifférence* 107, 112
benzodiazepine dependence
    in panic disorder 35
    predisposing factors 39, 60
    in somatization disorder 100
benzodiazepines
    in adjustment disorders 131
    in agoraphobia 56
    amnesic effects 131
    in generalized anxiety
        disorder 20, 39, 146
    in panic disorder 39
    in somatization disorder 93
bereavement
    as a mental disorder 77
beta-adrenergic blocking drugs
    in acute stress reactions 60
    in agoraphobia 56, 60–1
    in generalized anxiety
        disorder 40
    in panic disorder 40, 60
    in social phobia 61

biofeedback 38
bipolar (affective) disorders 64, 70
blindness 99, 106
blocking
    of panic attacks 19, 37, 57
blushing
    in social phobia 45–6
bodily symptoms
    differentiation of organic and
        psychological causes 110
    in depressive disorders 64, 66–8
    in dissociative disorders 110
    in generalized anxiety
        disorder 26–7
    in hypochondriasis 96–7, 101
    in panic attacks 18–20, 33
    in panic disorder 22–3
    in somatoform disorders 98–100,
        102, 110
body dysmorphic disorder 91, 95–6
borderline personality
    disorder 108, 128
    classification 9
borderline personality
    syndrome 158–60
Briquet's syndrome 92, 101, 115–6
bulimia nervosa 4–5
buspirone 40

cancer phobia 42–3
catastrophising theory
    in panic disorder 39
chest pain
    in panic disorder 22
choking sensations
    in panic disorder 22
chronic neurosis 150
claustrophobia 52
clomipramine
    efficacy 58–60
    in obsessive–compulsive
        disorder 58
cognitions
    in panic disorder 38
cognitive therapy
    in agoraphobia with panic 61–2
    in depressive disorders 81–5

in generalized anxiety
    disorder 82–4
in panic disorder 31, 82–4
co-morbidity of neurotic
    disorders 133–5
compulsions
    distinction between 50
    in general neurotic
        syndrome 156
    in obsessive–compulsive
        neurosis 50–1
concentration difficulty
    in depresive disorders 65–8
    in generalized anxiety
        disorder 27
congruence of mood in depressive
    disorders 66–8
conversion hysteria 91, 106–7, 111–2
cothymia 152–3
counselling 146
cueing
    in development of
        agoraphobia 32
cyclothymia 70

deafness 99
delusional disorder 96
delusions
    in depressive disorder 66–8, 148
dementia 75
dependence
    on alprazolam 60
    on benzodiazepines 35–9, 56
    on MAOIs 56
dependent personality disorder
    in anxiety disorders 137, 149
    classification 8
    in general neurotic
        syndrome 156–60
depersonalization–derealization
    syndrome 105, 112
depersonalization disorder 105, 112
depression
    in general neurotic
        syndrome 155
depressive illness, *see also*
    dysthymia, major depressive
    episode *and* melancholia

and adjustment disorders 122
in obsessive–compulsive
disorder 55
in panic disorder 32–3
outcome 137
and somatoform disorders 113
treatment 80–6
depressive neurosis, *see also*
dysthymia
classification 3–4, 63–4, 73–4
and depressive psychosis 64
depressive personality 70
depressive psychosis 64, 66–8,
77–8, 80–1, *see also* severe
depressive episode
desensitization 56–7
dexamethasone suppression
test 77
diagnostic consistency
of Briquet's syndrome 115–6
of hysteria 116
of stress and adjustment
disorders 127
diagnostic guidelines in ICD-10 4
*Diagnostic and Statistical Manual of
Mental Disorders* 10, 13–16
diarrhoea, *see* gastrointestinal
symptoms
diazepam
in dissociative disorders 94
in dysthymia 82–4
in GAD 82–4
in panic 82–4
dieting 5
disease phobias, *see* nosophobia
dissociative disorder
case history 93–4
classification 2, 88
description 103–9
overlap 111–5
stability 142
treatment 117
dizziness
in general neurotic
syndrome 154
in generalized anxiety
disorder 27, 136
in panic disorder 21, 22

in cognitive therapy 38
in somatization disorder 98–9
diurnal mood swing 65–8
dothiepin 82–4
double depression 75
DSM-III-R, *see Diagnostic and
Statistical Manual of Mental
Disorders*
dysmorphophobia, *see* body
dysmorphic disorder
dyspnoea
in general neurotic
syndrome 154
in generalized anxiety
disorder 27
in panic disorder 22
in somatization disorder 98–9
dysthymia
case history 69
classification 64, 71
and major depressive
episodes 72–3
primary and secondary 71–2
outcome 76–8
overlap 75–6
stability 142

early morning waking 65–8
eating disorders 3, 4–5
electroconvulsive therapy (ECT)
81
electrolyte disturbances 114
emotionally unstable personality
disorder 9, 10
endogenous anxiety 29
epidemic hysteria 108, 116
epilepsy 99, 107, 116
episodic paroxysmal anxiety, *see*
panic disorder
exercise
as form of treatment 38
exposure therapy
in agoraphobia 57–9
compared with other
psychological
treatments 61–2
duration of effects 58–9
to internal symptoms 38–9, 61–2

exposure therapy (*cont.*)
  in obsessive–compulsive
    disorder 57–9
  in post-traumatic stress
    disorder 130
  self-treatment 85
  in simple phobia 46–7, 56, 59
  in social phobia 59
eyelid twitch
  in generalized anxiety
    disorder 26

facial dyskinesia 106
factitious psychosis 89
family studies 138–9, 162
fatiguability
  in depressive disorders 66–8, 71
  in generalized anxiety
    disorder 26
fatigue, *see also* neurasthenia 26–7
fear
  in panic disorder 18, 19, 23
  reasonable and
    unreasonable 51–2
flashbacks 124
flushes
  in panic disorder 23
fluvoxamine 60
free-floating anxiety, *see* unfocused
  anxiety
fugue, *see* psychogenic fugue

GAD, *see* generalized anxiety
  disorder
Ganser symptoms 109
Ganser syndrome 105, 108–9
gastrointestinal symptoms
  in generalized anxiety
    disorder 17, 26–7
  in panic disorder 23
  in somatization disorder 93,
    98–9
gene locus
  for panic 29
general neurotic syndrome
  classification 152
  description 133
  identification 153–60

personality in 156–9
  symptom change 155
General Neurotic Syndrome Scale
  (GNSS) 159
generalized anxiety disorder
  case history 24–5
  classification 26–7
  description 20
  differences from panic
    disorder 22–7
  drug treatment 39–40, 82–4
  genetic effects 160–2
  origin of diagnosis 20
  outcome 30–7
  overlap 29–30
  and panic disorder 17–41
  psychological treatment 38–40
  reliability 28–9
  stability 142
genetic influences
  in anxiety–depressive (mixed)
    disorder 160–2
  in generalized anxiety
    disorder 29, 160–2
  in panic disorder 29, 160–2
globus hystericus 111
guilt
  in depressive disorders 65

hallucinations
  in depressive disorders 66–8
  in post-traumatic stress
    disorder 125
haloperidol 38
headache 27, 154
hierarchy
  of classification of neurotic
    disorders 133–41
  in panic disorder 30
histrionic personality disorder
  and adjustment disorders 128
  classification 8
  and somatoform disorders 114–5
hopelessness 66–7, 71
5-hydroxytryptamine (5-HT) 59
  reuptake inhibitors 59–60
hypersensitivity to rejection 29
hypersomnia 3, 5–6, 66–7, 71

hyperventilation
  aetiology 33–4
  in treatment of panic disorder 38
hypochondriacal personality
  disorder 115
hypochondriasis
  in generalized anxiety
    disorder 33–4
  in panic disorder 33
  as a primary disorder 91, 96–7,
    101
  and somatization disorder 34
  and somatoform disorders 113
  in schizophrenia 96
hysteria
  classification 88
  definition 86–7
  and organic disorders 90, 114
  outcome 90–2
  social aspects 109
hysterical hypochondriasis 101
hysterical pseudodementia, see
  Ganser syndrome
hysterical psychosis 88, 94
hysterical stupor 107
hysteroepilepsy 116

identity disturbance 108
illusions 125
imipramine
  in agoraphobia 58–9
  anti-panic vs anti-phobic
    effects 57
  dosage and response 38
  in panic disorder 19–20, 37
impulsive personality disorder 128
insomnia
  in depressive disorders 65–8, 71
  in generalized anxiety
    disorder 26–7
  in post-traumatic stress
    disorder 124–6
  as primary disorder 3
interest, lack of
  in depressive disorders 65–9
  in post-traumatic stress
    disorder 126
International Classification of

Disease (ICD) 1–12
interview schedules
  for mental state 156–8
  for personality disorder 157-60
irritability
  in anxiety neurosis 17
  in generalized anxiety
    disorder 27
  jealousy
  morbid 50

Kleine Levin syndrome 5–6

lability
  emotional 136–7
lactate injections
  in treatment of anxiety 39
life events
  in adjustment disorders 128–9
  in anxiety 150
  in depression 150
  in obesity 4–5
  in personality disorders 128
  in somatization disorder 93

major depressive episode
  and anxiety disorders 75–6
  case history 69
  classification 64–8, 134
  outcome 76–8
  overlap with other depressive
    disorders 73–6
  and panic disorder 32–3
  stability 142
  treatment 67, 80–6
malingering 89, 107, 110
mania 63–4
melancholia 65
mild depressive episodes
  classification 68
  outcome 76–80
  overlap 74–6
  treatment 80–5
mitral valve prolapse 35
mixed neurotic syndromes 132
  see also anxiety–depressive
    (mixed) disorder and general
    neurotic syndrome

monoamine oxidase inhibitors
(MAOIs)
in agoraphobia 56, 60, 146
in depressive disorders 81
in generalized anxiety
disorder 60–1
in obsessive–compulsive
disorder 60
in panic disorder 56, 146
in social phobia 60, 146
spectrum of efficacy 61
monosymptomatic
hypochondriacal psychosis 96
monosymptomatic phobia, *see*
simple phobia
motor tension
in general neurotic
syndrome 154
in generalized anxiety
disorder 26
in hypochondriasis 101
multiple personality disorder
104–6, 112
muscle aches
in general neurotic
syndrome 154
in generalized anxiety
disorder 26
in somatization disorder 98–9
muscle tension, *see* motor tension

narcissistic personality disorder 9,
128
narcolepsy 5–6
nausea 23, 27, 98, 154
neurasthenia 2, 17
neurosis
definition 11
in DSM-III 13–16
neurotic character 7, 149
neurotic traits in childhood 137
new antidepressants 56, 59–60
nightmares 3, 124
nihilism 66–7
nortriptyline 60
nosophobia 42, 43, 97
numbness
emotional 124–6

obesity 3, 4–5, 25
obsessional symptoms
in depressive disorders 50
obsessive–compulsive disorder
(neurosis)
case history 47
classification 2, 51, 134
description 50
outcome 55–6
overlap 54
relapse 56
stability 55, 142
treatment 56–60
obsessive–compulsive personality
disorder, *see* anankastic
personality disorder
Oedipus complex 90
oral personality, *see* dependent
personality disorder
outcome, *see also individual named
diagnoses*
of acute stress reactions 129
of adjustment disorder 129–30
of post-traumatic stress
disorder 129–30

pain 98, 102–3
palpitations
in general neurotic
syndrome 154
in panic disorder 21, 22
in somatization disorder 92,
98–9
panic attacks
case history 21–2
and conversion hysteria 34
definition 21
and depersonalization 112
derivation 19
description by Freud 17–18
in general neurotic
syndrome 154
reliability 25
situational 20–1, 28
spontaneous 19–20, 28, 32, 34
in stress and adjustment
disorders 31, 128

panic disorder
  blocking by drugs  19, 37, 57
  case history  21–4
  classification  21, 22–3
  definition  21, 22–3
  distinction from generalized
    anxiety disorder  145–8
  genetic factors  160–2
  and hypochondriasis  34–5
  limited symptom attacks  23
  mortality  35
  prevalence  31
  outcome  30–7, 55
  overlap  29–30
  reliability  25–6, 28
  spontaneous vs situational  28
  stability  142
  treatment  37–41
paraesthesias
  in anxiety  17–8
  in panic disorder  23
paralysis  88, 99, 103, 111
paranoid personality disorder  8
parasuicide  119
paroxysmal hemicrania  106
passive–aggressive personality
    disorder  9
perception
  dissociation of  105, 108
pernicious anaemia  135
personality
  dissociation of  103, 104–6
personality change  106
personality disorder, *see also*
    multiple personality disorder
  in adjustment disorders  128–9
  in chronic neurotic disorder  55
  classification  3
  in depressive disorders  66–8
  and dissociative disorders  114–5
  historical aspects  7–8
  and neurotic disorder  9–10,
    149–50
  and somatoform disorders  114–5
pharmacological dissection  37,
    85–6
phenelzine  60
phobic avoidance, *see* avoidance

phobic disorders
  alcohol and drug dependence  55
  as anxiety states  52
  classification  2, 42–4
  and depersonalization  108
  Klein's views of origin  19–20
  outcome  55–6
  overlap  54
  personality status  150
  relapse  56
  stability  141–2
  treatment  56–62
porphyria  114
possession states  103, 108
post-traumatic stress disorder
  case history  119–20
  description  124–6
  differential diagnosis  129
  outcome  129–30
  overlap  128–9
  prevalence  121–2
  reliability  127
  stability  142
  treatment  130–1
premenstrual tension syndrome  3
primary care  149–50
psychoanalysis
  and classification  14–5
  origin of  90
psychogenic amnesia  88, 98–9,
    104, 107, 112, 126
psychogenic fugue  88, 103, 104, 112
psychomotor retardation
  in depressive disorders  64–8
psychophysiological changes
  in anxiety  151
  in depression  151
  in panic  20
psychoses
  definition  11
psychosocial stressors
  and adjustment disorders
    118–20, 122
  and dissociative disorders  88,
    93–5, 103–9
  in general neurotic
    syndrome  155
  in hysteria  87–8

psychotherapy
and classification of
neuroses 14–16, 163
group 130
in generalized anxiety 38–40
in neuroses 145–6
in post-traumatic stress
disorder 130–1
in stress and adjustment
disorders 130
interpersonal 81

relaxation 25
response prevention
in obsessive–compulsive
disorder 47
restlessness in generalized anxiety
disorder 26–27
retardation, *see* psychomotor
retardation
ruminations 51

sadistic personality disorder 10
Schedule for Affective Disorders
and Schizophrenia 156
schizoaffective disorder 64–5, 75
schizoid personality disorder 8,
149
schizophrenia
classification 135
and depressive disorders 75
and hysteria 116
and obsessional disorder 55
schizotypal personality disorder 8
secondary gain 88, 103
self-defeating personality
disorder 10
self-help treatment 82–4
separation anxiety 20, 52–3
severe depressive episode
classification 64–8
outcome 65
treatment 65
sex incidence
in agoraphobia 52
in epidemic hysteria 116
in somatization disorder 102, 115

sexual dysfunctions
classification 3
in somatization disorder 99–100
shortness of breath, *see* dyspnoea
simple phobia
antidepressant drugs in 49
case history 46–7
classification 43
description 49–50
natural history 49
treatment 56
sleep, *see* sleep disorder,
hypersomnia *and* insomnia
sleep disorder 3, 5–6
snake phobia 46–7, 53
social adjustment 60, 100, 122, 135
social phobia
case history 45–6
definition 43, 48–9
overlap 54
and panic disorder 36, 49
treatment 60–1
somatization
in affective disorder 113
in anxiety 113
somatization disorder
case history 92–3
classification 91, 98–9
depression and 99
onset 102
and panic attacks 34
psychotherapy 93
somatoform disorders
classification 2, 88, 91
definition 89
overlap 111–5
stability 142
somatoform pain disorder 91,
102–3
spastic oesophagus 106
specific phobia, *see* simple phobia
spontaneous panics, *see* panic
attacks
stability
of diagnosis 134, 141–3
startle response 124–6
stress, *see* acute stress disorder *and*
psychosocial stressors

stupor 103
subclinical neurosis 152–3
suicide
    in panic disorder 35
swallowing
    difficulty in 27, 98–9
sweating
    in general neurotic
        syndrome 154
    in generalized anxiety
        disorder 27
    in panic disorder 23
symtoms
    and diagnosis 133–4
systemic lupus erythematosus 114

temperaments
    in depressive disorders 77
thioridazine 93
thoracic outlet syndrome 106
time course
    of neuroses 143–5
tingling sensations, see
    paraesthesias
torticollis 106
trance states 104
transexualism 108
trembling
    in general neurotic
        syndrome 154
    in generalized anxiety
        disorder 26
    in panic disorder 23
tricyclic antidepressants, see
    antidepressants
twilight states 109

twin studies of neurotic
    disorder 29, 160–2

unconscious motivation 87–9
undifferentiated somatoform
    disorder 91, 102
unfocused anxiety 17, 20
unreality feelings
    in panic disorder 23
urinary symptoms
    in general neurotic
        syndrome 154
    in generalized anxiety
        disorder 27
    in somatization disorder 99

venereal disease
    phobia of 43
vertigo 17
visual disturbance 98–9
voice loss 98–9
vomiting
    in eating disorders 3, 5
    phobias of 49, 53
    in somatization disorder 98–9
*Vorbeireden* 109
vulnerability 129–30

war neurosis 90, 112
weight loss
    in depressive disorders 65–8, 151
whiplash syndrome 106–7
wind phobia 50
World Health Organization 1
worthlessness
    in depressive disorders 65–9
writer's cramp 107